THE RESPIRATORY ROLE OF THE UPPER AIRWAYS

A SELECTIVE CLINICAL AND PATHOPHYSIOLOGICAL REVIEW

THE RESPIRATORY ROLE OF THE UPPER AIRWAYS

A SELECTIVE CLINICAL AND PATHOPHYSIOLOGICAL REVIEW

PHILIP COLE, M.D., F.R.C.S.(C)
The University Departments of Otolaryngology
St. Michael's Hospital
Hospital for Sick Children
The Gage Research Institute
Toronto, Canada

Mosby Year Book

St. Louis Baltimore Boston Chicago London Philadelphia Sydney Toronto

Mosby Year Book

Dedicated to Publishing Excellence

Sponsoring Editor: James D. Ryan
Assistant Director, Manuscript Services: Frances M. Perveiler
Senior Production Assistant: Maria Nevinger
Proofroom Manager: Barbara M. Kelly

Mosby–Year Book, Inc.
11830 Westline Industrial Drive
St. Louis, MO 63146

1 2 3 4 5 6 7 8 9 0 GW MV 97 96 95 94 93

Library of Congress Cataloging-in-Publication Data

Cole, Philip.
The respiratory role of the upper airways: a selective clinical and pathophysiological review / Philip Cole.
p. cm.
Includes bibliographical references and index.
ISBN 1-55664-390-X
1. Nose—Diseases. 2. Throat—Diseases. 3. Respiratory organs—Diseases. I. Title.
[DNLM: 1. Nasal Obstruction—physiopathology. 2. Respiration—physiology. 3. Respiration Disorders—physiopathology. WF 102 C689r]
RF341.C65 1992 92-19173
616.2—dc20 CIP
DNLM/DLC
for Library of Congress

For Raya

FOREWORD

My old friend, the late Sven Ingelstedt of Lund, Sweden, first turned my attention to the work of Philip Cole. At the time I thought of Ingelstedt as the world leader in upper airway physiology, and Ingelstedt thought of Cole in the same light. During the decades since then I have learned how right Ingelstedt was. Philip Cole is without doubt the world leader in upper airway physiology and its application to otolaryngology, especially in relation to problems of air pollution.

We are indeed fortunate to have a text from his hand. To my mind it is particularly gratifying to note that Cole has viewed the upper airway as a whole, the extrathoracic airway. He also has carried out the definitive work on the relative role of the nasopharyngeal and oropharyngeal paths of airflow. And, finally, he has seen that a major role of the nose is its efficacy in defense of the lungs.

In summary, I suggest to all those with an abiding and penetrating curiosity about any phase of respiratory function and disease that they will be well rewarded by study and enjoyment of this unique volume. I am proud to call Philip my friend and am delighted to congratulate him on an important job very well done.

DONALD F. PROCTOR, M.D.
Emeritus Professor
Environmental Health Sciences
The Johns Hopkins Medical Institutions
Baltimore, Maryland

PREFACE

This book was written by an otolaryngologist as a companion to general ENT texts and although directed primarily toward clinicians, in training and in practice, it contains material that will be new and useful to others interested in respirology of the upper airways.

Knowledge of respiratory function and dysfunction of the airways outside the lungs, traditionally the clinical territory of the otolaryngologist, has been enriched in recent years by contributions from several clinical specialties and basic sciences. Recognition of breathing disorders in sleep has provided a stimulus for an explosion of publications concerned with respiratory function of these airways.

The focus of this book is on respiratory function. Current topics that are widely scattered throughout several biomedical fields and as yet incompletely incorporated in general ENT texts have been chosen for their clinical importance and physiological interest. Repetition of material that is comprehensively covered in these texts has been minimized and used only to amplify or clarify the subject under discussion.

The nose, mouth, and pharynx comprise a complex of air passages at the entrance to the respiratory tract whose primary role is to serve and protect the lower airways. Although the lumen of these extra-pulmonary passages is termed "dead space" by pulmonary respirologists, it consists of lively segments that conduct, resist, and limit flow of respiratory air. Sites, functions, and dysfunctions of these segments in the nasal, oral, and pharyngeal airways are discussed in the following chapters. Their respiratory roles in awake and sleeping subjects together with the palatal switching mechanism and nose/mouth breathing are examined. The modification of air in the respiratory passages is described and a critical discussion of symptomatology, clinical assessment, and methods of objective measurement of nasal, oral, and pharyngeal respiratory function are presented in the concluding chapter.

It is the author's intent that this selective review will assist in decision-making by otolaryngologists, who, in addition to treating traditional ENT diseases, are increasingly involved in the management of such diverse disorders as those concerned with breathing in sleep, orthodontics, and allergy. It is hoped also that others who are faced with the ubiquitous clinical problems associated with the upper air passages will find this volume helpful.

PHILIP COLE M.D., F.R.C.S.(C)

ACKNOWLEDGMENTS

The manuscript from which this textbook has been produced is based on the work of many investigators and clinicians in addition to my colleagues, fellows, and associates in the Departments of Otolaryngology and Respirology and the Gage Research Institute, University of Toronto. I am grateful to all including the many whose work is not acknowledged in the reference sections of the text.

I offer my thanks also to Dr. Ronald Eccles, Cardiff, Professor Noe Zamel, Toronto, Professor Peter A.R. Clement, Brussels, and Dr. Victor Hirsch, Royal Palm Beach, Florida, for their helpful comments on early drafts of Chapters 1 to 4.

PHILIP COLE, M.D., F.R.C.S.(C)

CONTENTS

CHAPTER 1

The Nose

NASAL RESPIRATORY FUNCTION

Introduction

In many animal species the nose is a prominent and complex organ with an extensive olfactory mucosa and a turbinate structure that achieves exotic proliferation. By contrast, in humans the olfactory mucosa is restricted to a relatively small area and the turbinates are vestigial.[32] The area of human olfactory mucosa is a half, and turbinate mucosa a quarter, that of the domestic cat[134] (Figs 1–1 and 1–2).

Life can be sustained indefinitely without use of nasal airways by tracheostomal breathing.[89] Indeed, the human nose impedes respiratory airflow and, despite its reputation as an effective air cleanser and conditioner, it is bypassed by mouth breathing in the increased ventilatory response to exercise when air cleansing and conditioning demands are high.

As a conduit for $>12{,}000$ L/day of inspired ambient air weighing almost 15 kg, the nose is a portal of entry for gaseous and particulate noxious materials. It is the principal site of particle deposition from inspired air and a reservoir of pathogenic microorganisms. The nose carries a heavy burden of morbidity and is a major source of diseases that afflict all mankind.

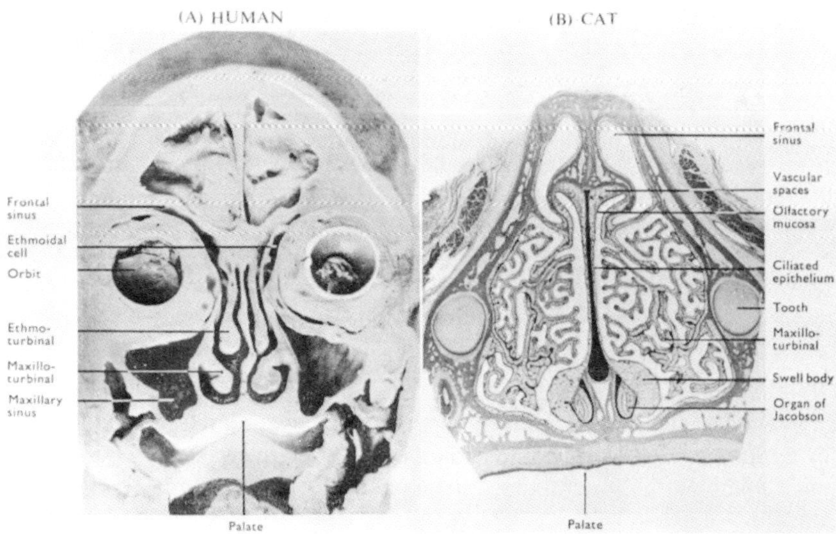

FIG 1–1.

Coronal sections. Comparison between human **(A)** and cat **(B)** nasal cavities. (From Negus VE: *The Comparative Anatomy and Physiology of the Nose and Paranasal Sinuses.* London, Churchill Livingstone, 1958, p 193. Used by permission.)

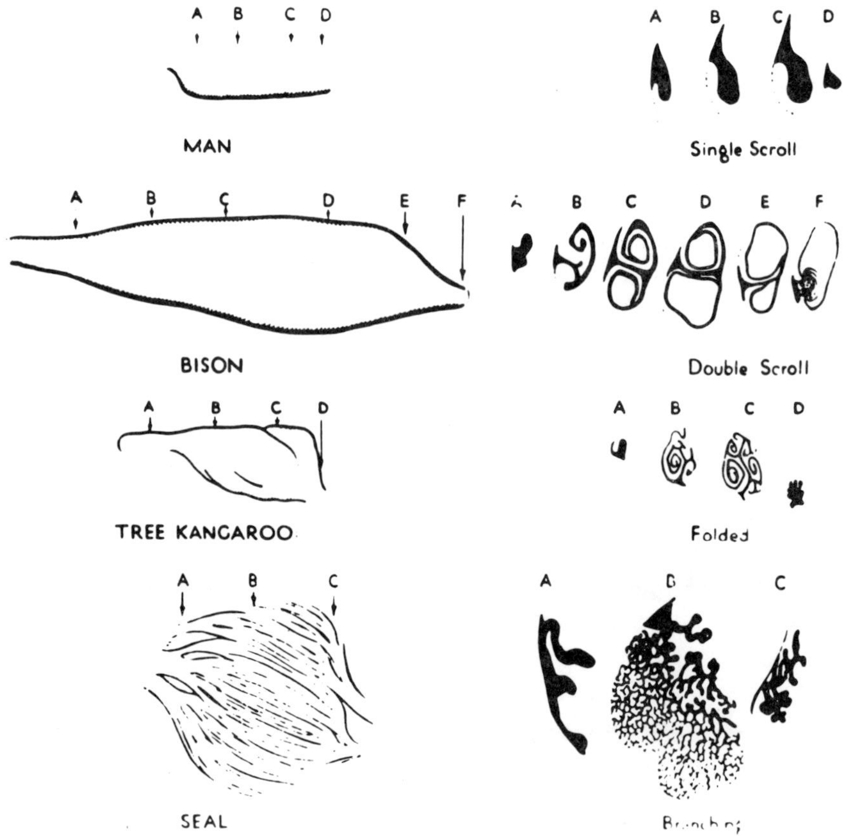

FIG 1–2.

Maxilloturbinals. Comparison between humans and animals. (From Negus VE: *The Comparative Anatomy and Physiology of the Nose and Paranasal Sinuses.* London, Churchill Livingstone, 1958, p 195. Used by permission.)

Nasal Breathing

Despite these negative attributes, the answer to Proctor's rhetorical question, "Is the human nose more than a vestigial olfactory organ?" is in the affirmative, and important roles of this relatively simple organ as a functioning or malfunctioning participant in the respiratory process are described in this volume. The principal nasal components that regulate respiratory airflow—the structural narrowing of the nasal valve and the lumen-regulating erectile mucosa—are discussed in detail in this chapter.

The healthy nose provides a preferential breathing route, yet, in comparison with other segments of the breathing passages, its resistance to respiratory airflow is high. In fact, the major single component of resistance of the entire respiratory tract is localized to a specific anterior nasal segment a few millimeters in length[76] (Figs 1–3 to 1–6). Combined resistances of the short, narrowed segments at each nasal portal approach the magnitude of the combined resistances of the remainder of the nasal airways of each side,

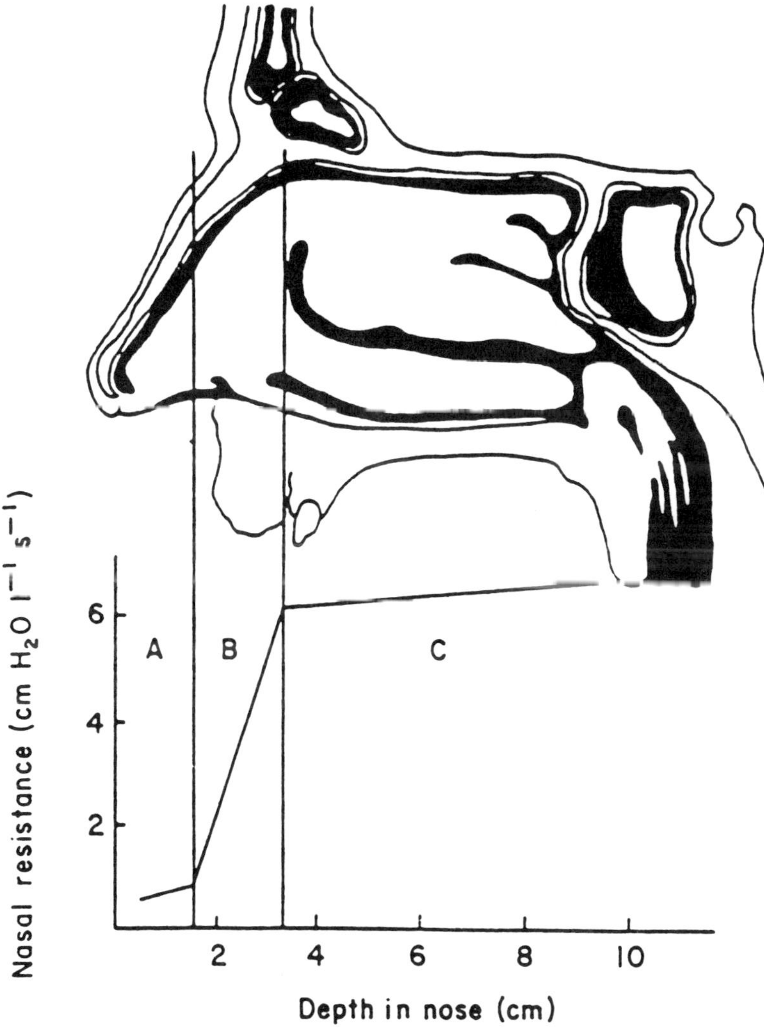

FIG 1–3.

Diagrammatic divisions of a nasal cavity: **A,** vestibular entrance; **B,** resistive valve region; **C,** minimally resistive cavum. (From Eccles R: Rhinomanometry and nasal challenge, in Mackay IS, Bull TR (eds): *Scott Brown's Otolaryngology,* ed 5. London, Butterworth, 1987, p 41. Used by permission.)

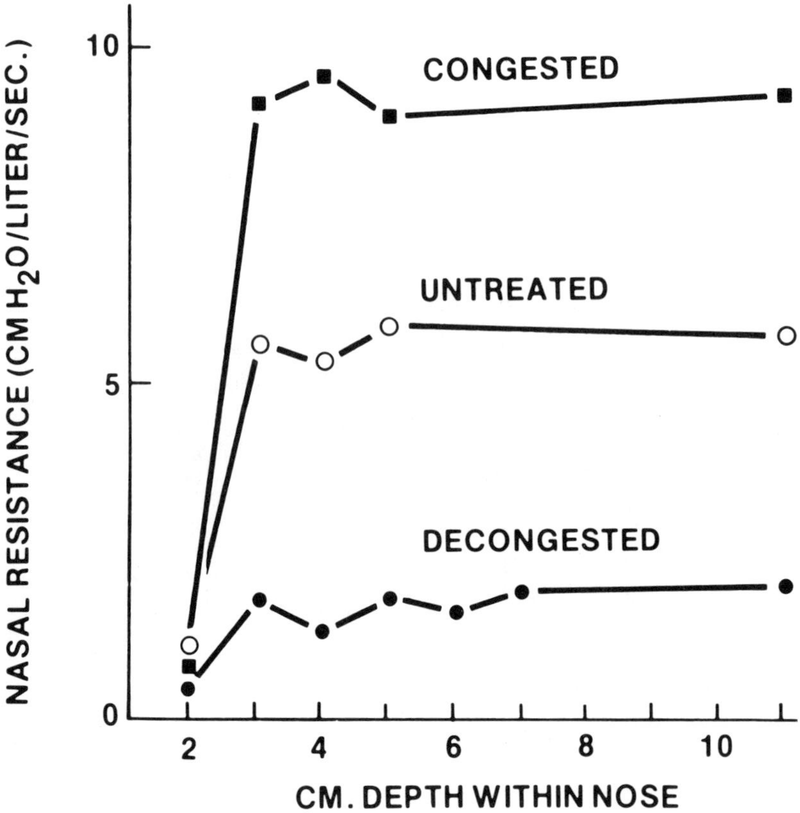

FIG 1–4.

Measured nasal resistances at sites within a nasal cavity. Resistance is localized at 2 to 3 cm in the congested, untreated, and decongested mucosal state. There is little resistance change in cavum between 3 and 10 cm. (From Haight JSJ, Cole P: The site and function of the nasal valve. *Laryngoscope* 1983; 93(1):49. Used by permission.)

together with the pharynx, larynx, trachea, bronchi, and the peripheral pulmonary airways.

The nostril, shaped and supported by the lower alar cartilage, provides access to the nasal vestibule. The vestibular lumen converges to a triangular slit bounded laterally by the caudal end of the upper alar cartilage and medially by the septum. The sides of the triangle meet at an acute apical angle of $<15°$ and its short base lies across the floor of the nose (Figs 1–7 and 1–8). These boundaries define the entrance to the nasal valve, an entrance that is obliquely situated between the horizontal nostril and the vertical piriform aperture. The lumen of the valve is oblique also in relation to the median sagittal plane from which it diverges slightly to enter the cavum.

THE NASAL VALVE

Description

Sites of narrowing and resistance to airflow in the anterior nose are variously described in the literature. At least ten different terms, several of them synonymous, confuse descriptions of this region.[100] Writers seldom emphasize that in addition to the resistive importance of its cross-sectional dimensions,[9] the nasal valve is a dynamic segment of the airway. It has a length of several millimeters, and its lumen follows a much longer and narrower course dorsally than ventrally. This segment[44, 172] extends from its triangular entrance, described above, to the piriform region of the cavum.[150]

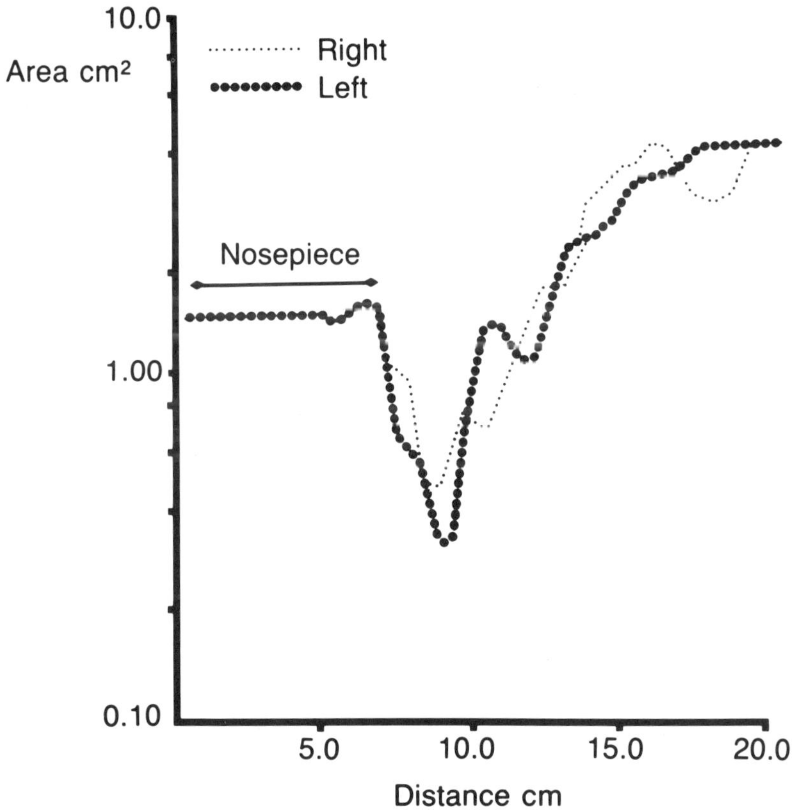

FIG 1–5.

Cross-sectional areas (log scale) of nasal cavity measured by acoustic reflection. (From Hilberg AC, Swift DZ, Pedersen OF: Acoustic rhinometry: Evaluation of nasal cavity geometry by acoustic reflection. *J Appl Physiol* 1989; 66(1):295. Used by permission.)

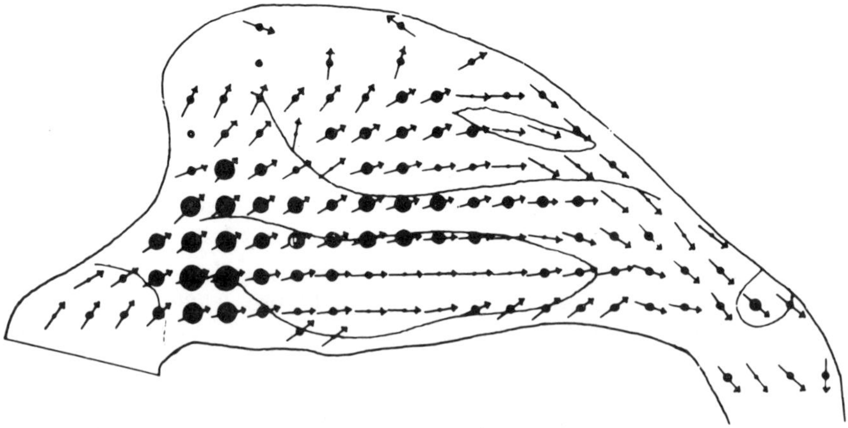

FIG 1–6.
Measured linear velocities and directions of the inspiratory airstream. Sizes of circles indicate velocity; arrows indicate direction. (From Swift DL, Proctor DF: Access of air to the respiratory tract, in Brain JD, Proctor DF, Reid LM (eds): *Respiratory Defense Mechanisms.* New York, Marcel Dekker, 1977, p 80. Used by permission.)

The nasal valve consists of the anterior bony cavum containing inferior turbinate erectile tissue, lateral-wall erectile tissue anterior to the turbinate, and septal erectile tissue, supported respectively by compliant alar tissues and the rigid cartilaginous septum. These elements combine to form a dynamic valve that adjusts nasal airflow. It is stabilized by cartilage and bone, modulated by voluntary muscles, and regulated by erectile tissues.

Airflow

There are marked inter-subject and inter-racial differences in configuration and airflow resistances of this region of the nose (Figs 1–9 and 1–10). This subject is discussed further in the section on "Nasal Airway Stability" in Chapter 4. Here the airstream makes a right-angle turn around the short sector of the nasal floor between nostril and piriform aperture as the mainstream of air flows through the basal portion of the valve. The essential physiologic role of the nasal valve in the respiratory process is examined in Chapter 3.

Voluntary facial muscles assist in stabilizing the compliant alae against transmural pressures generated by inspiratory airflow (see next section of this chapter, "Alar Compliance"), and these muscles also shape facial expressions that signify emotions such as disgust, fear, and anger. Furthermore, muscular positioning of the alae directs the inspiratory airstream as a thin (2 to 3 mm width) ribbon to an arched course along the septum between the superior and inferior turbinates (see Fig 1–6) or alternatively, by olfactory sniffs, to the roof of the nose. The olfactory recess is sheltered from the main blast of unconditioned inspiratory air and is swept clear of ambient olfactants by widely dispersed and well conditioned expiratory air.[173] Sniffs can also be directed to clear mucus from the nasal cavities, snorts propel it to the pharynx, and inspiration through partially collapsed alae sucks mucus from sinus ostia.

A

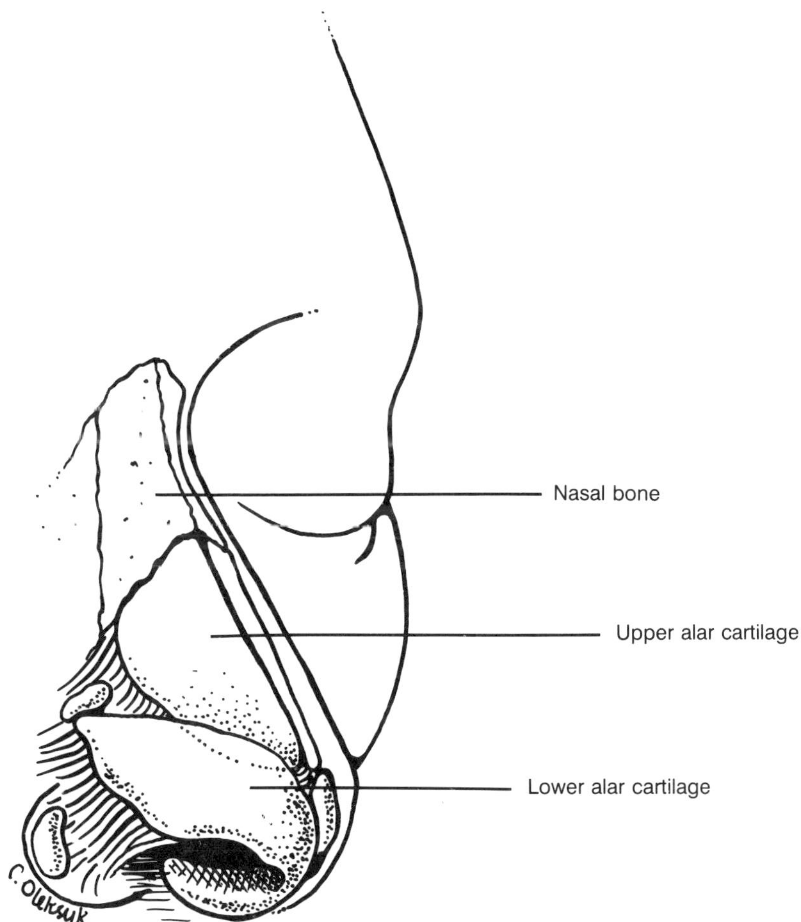

FIG 1–7.
A, nasal skeleton. *(Continued.)*

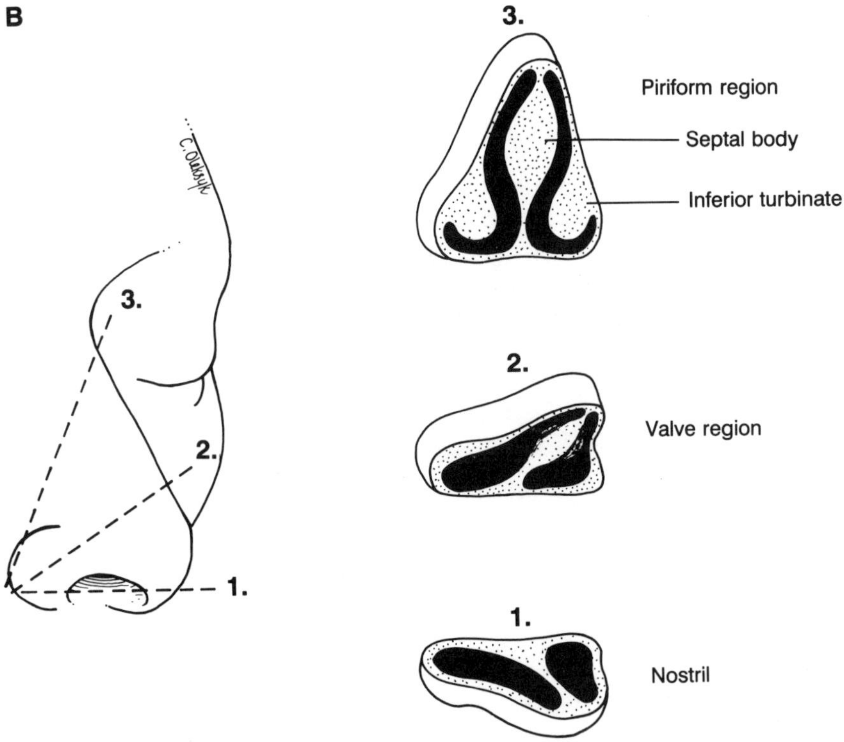

FIG 1-7 (cont.).
B, lumen of anterior nose.

Lumen Dimensions

In recent years cadaver, model, and cast studies[173, 9] have demonstrated the small cross-sectional dimensions of the Caucasian nasal valve, the narrow but more roomy cavum (Table 1–1; also see Figs 1–1 to 1–6 and 1–21 to 1–25), and intrusion on the airway by erectile tissues superimposed on the structural lumen of the nose (see Figs 1–7 and 1–8). These studies confirm observations made many decades ago,[52, 125, 196] and they are further substantiated by the most recent in vivo investigations by acoustic reflection[70, 113] (see Fig 1–5) as well as by computer-assisted airflow measurements[76, 94] (see Fig 1–3).

Clinical comment: The nasal valve is the principal respiratory airflow resistor of the entire breathing tract. It is stabilized by cartilage and bone, modulated by voluntary muscles, and regulated by erectile tissues.

ALAR COMPLIANCE

Transmural Pressures

Alar compliance with inspiratory transmural pressures is restricted by attachments of the alar cartilages, by resistance to deformation of alar tissues, and by isometric, inspiratory, alar dilator muscle contractions.[117, 157, 158, 53] However, although respiratory alar movement is seldom seen in adult humans during tidal breathing at rest, small inspiratory movements of the less restricted caudal end of the upper alar cartilage toward the septum have been detected on video studies of exercising subjects.[38] In addition, animal investigations have demonstrated transitory nasal mucosal decongestion with each inspiration that might compensate for inspiratory narrowing by alar movement.[57]

Alar Muscle Activity

Electromyographic studies show alar dilator muscle activity to accompany each nasal inspiration (Fig 1–11); it varies directly with ventilation, nasal

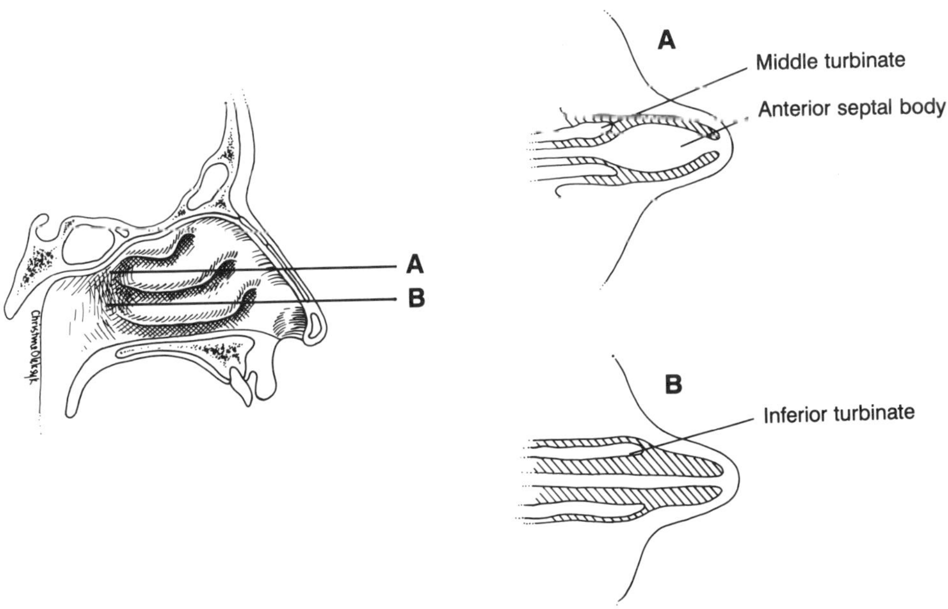

FIG 1–8.
A and **B,** diagrammatic sagittal view of lateral nasal wall and axial sections. Note septal body above the inferior turbinate and anterior to the middle turbinate.

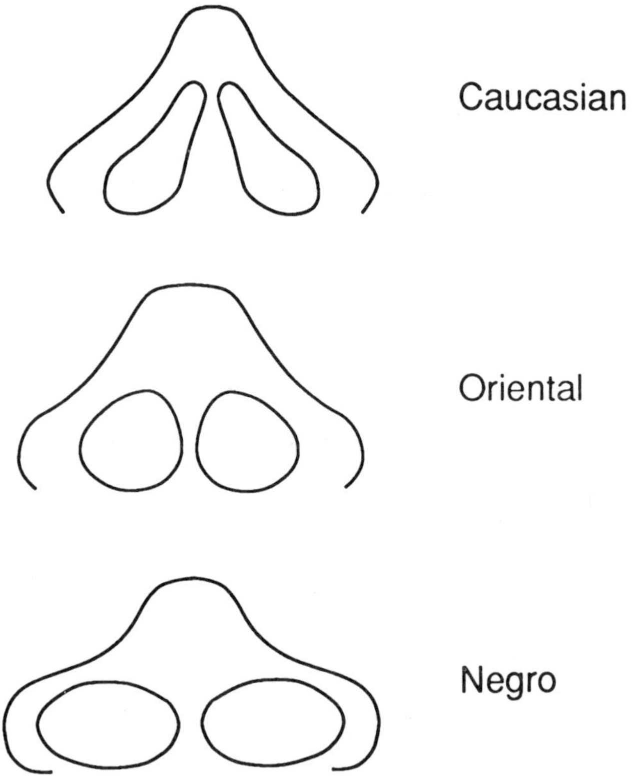

FIG 1–9.

Nostril shapes. (From Ohki M, Naito K, Cole P: Dimensions and resistances of the human nose. *Laryngoscope* 1991; 101(3):276. Used by permission.)

resistance, hypoxia, and hypercapnia and ceases with mouth or tracheostomal breathing.[157, 38] As with other upper-airway stabilizing muscles, this activity precedes diaphragmatic contraction.[118, 170] Recovery of alar muscle activity on resumption of use of the natural airway following lengthy periods of tracheostomal breathing is delayed or incomplete.[158, 157]

Alar muscle respiratory activity is directed not only toward stabilizing the anterior nasal airway but also toward increasing its patency as the situation demands. Spontaneous respiratory alar movement is not unusual in the young child even at rest but is seldom seen in adults. Adult alar muscle activity produces visible alar dilation only under exceptionally demanding conditions.

As airflow is maintained through a narrowed airway segment, linear velocity of the airstream increases and elevates transmural pressure, a compressing force, at the site of narrowing (Bernoulli). At a critical

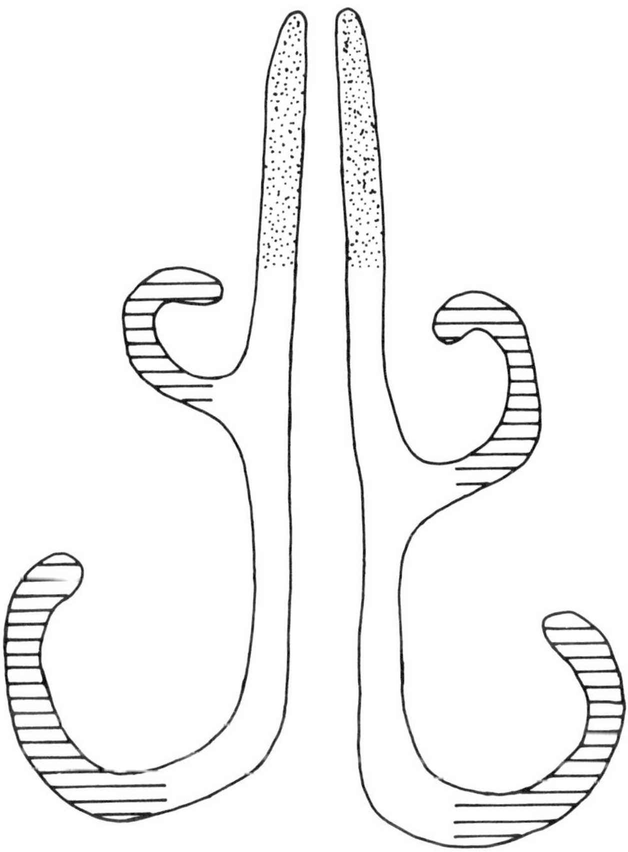

FIG 1–10.

Mid-caval lumen. *Unshaded area* = main nasal airway; *stippled area* = olfactory region; *hatched area* = meatuses. (From Proctor DF: The upper airway, in Proctor DF, Anderson I (eds): *The Nose: Upper Airway Physiology and the Atmospheric Environment.* Amsterdam, Elsevier Biomedical Press, 1982, p 28. Used by permission.)

TABLE 1–1.

Nasal Dimensions

Valve cross section	50 mm^2
Cavum cross section	150 mm^2
Airway width	1–3 mm
Width of meatuses	½–1 mm
Floor to cribriform plate	5 cm
Tip to posterior pharyngeal wall	11 cm
Mucosal area	150 cm^2
Volume	15 cm^3

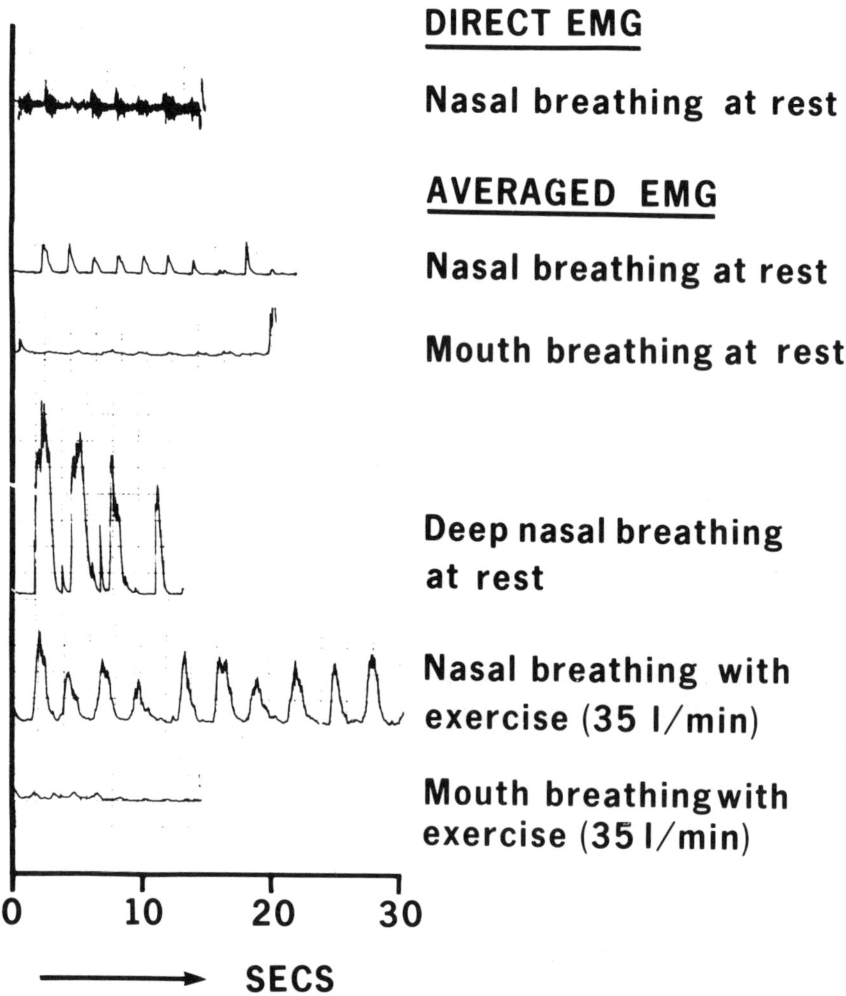

FIG 1–11.

Alar electromyograms. Amplitude increases with ventilation, and electrical activity ceases with mouth breathing. (From Cole P, Haight JSJ, Love L, et al: Dynamic components of nasal resistance. *Am Rev Respir Dis* 1985; 132:1229. Used by permission.)

inspiratory transmural pressure, the compliant portion of the narrow nasal valve collapses partially or completely and thus limits or occludes the airway (Fig 1–12) – for example, with a strong sniff through a single nostril.[21, 22, 156] A Starling valve effect may occur as the compliant tissues respond to transmural pressures, but until a critical transmural pressure is achieved, normal alar tissues and dilator muscles provide sufficient rigidity to withstand deformation.

Thus, lumen and resistance of the normally functioning valve is little affected by the transmural pressures that are generated by nasal breathing at rest. The switch to oronasal breathing that accompanies exercise (see Chapter 2, "Mouth Breathing") reduces the nasal fraction of respiratory airflow and the alar burden of transmural pressure.

Some values of cross-sectional area[81] derived from trans-nasal pressure and flow studies have suggested inspiratory widening of the nasal lumen. Resistance calculations have suggested the opposite. Neither calculation is supported by direct observation or video studies, which have detected no alar movement in healthy adult noses during spontaneous breathing of subjects at rest.

Inspiratory Alar Collapse

Passive valvular collapse in response to inspiratory transmural pressures is seen in cases of Bell's and other facial-muscle palsies. Alar flaccidity alar deformity, or muscular weakness—brought about by trauma or occurring as

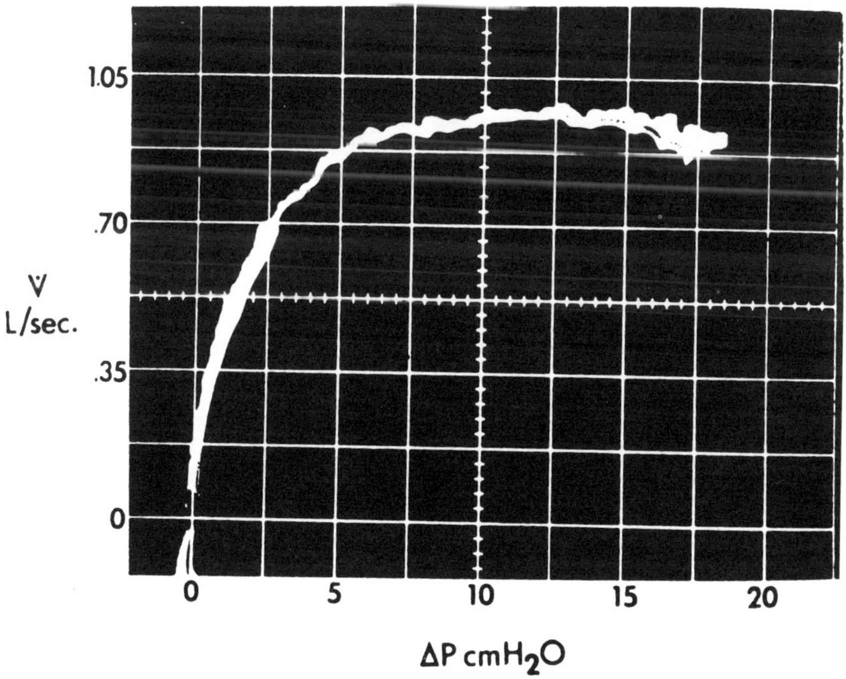

FIG 1–12.

Inspiratory flow limitation by partial alar collapse. (From Bridger GP: Physiology of the nasal valve. *Arch Otolaryngol* 1970; 92:543. Used by permission.)

complications of rhinoplasty[167, 51, 67] can each increase compliance and reduce the magnitude of the critical transmural closing pressure. Under these circumstances, partial or complete alar collapse and nasal obstruction can result from modest inspiratory airflow.

Inspiratory alar collapse is found frequently in association with ipsilateral narrowing caused by septal deviation. As flow of nasal inspiratory air maintains pulmonary ventilation, this pattern of alar malfunction is found also when transmural pressures are elevated by narrowing in the valve region caused by abnormalities of the alae, the mucosa, or a combination of these factors (Bernoulli).

The readiness with which inspiratory alar collapse can be brought about in healthy noses by a brisk sniff while the contralateral vestibule is occluded[22] suggests the possibility of alar dilator muscle inhibition. If such inhibition does take place on unilateral occlusion, resulting contralateral inspiratory narrowing could affect anterior rhinomanometric measurements (see Chapter 4, "Clinical Rhinomanometry").

Valve Patency

On average ($N = 100$) wide alar retraction reduces airflow resistance of the healthy Caucasian nose by about half. Topical decongestant then reduces it further to about one third of normal, while almost all remaining nasal resistance persists in the rigid caval entrance.[76] By contrast, in the absence of artificial interference with the narrow triangular confines of the nasal valve (for example, by a speculum), slight mucosal or skeletal intrusions on the lumen by the medial and/or lateral wall can result in substantial decrease in cross-sectional area and exponential increase in both airflow resistance and transmural pressure.

A small septal deformity or minor mucosal swelling in the anterior nose is a common cause of obstruction,[34, 28] whereas only gross deviations or swelling are obstructive in other parts of the nasal cavities (Figs 1–13 to 1–15). However, although an entirely regular midline septum in an adult is uncommon,[68, 180] septal irregularity is symptomless in most cases.

Trauma or buckling from disproportionate growth of skeletal facial structures are generally accepted explanations for the occurrence of septal deviations, which are found most frequently in adult males. There is evidence to support the view that they result also from parturition injuries sustained during rotation of the fetal head in the birth canal; and indeed, they are reported to be less frequent in cesarean than vaginal births.[68] A recent series cited 2% septal deviations in neonates.[61]

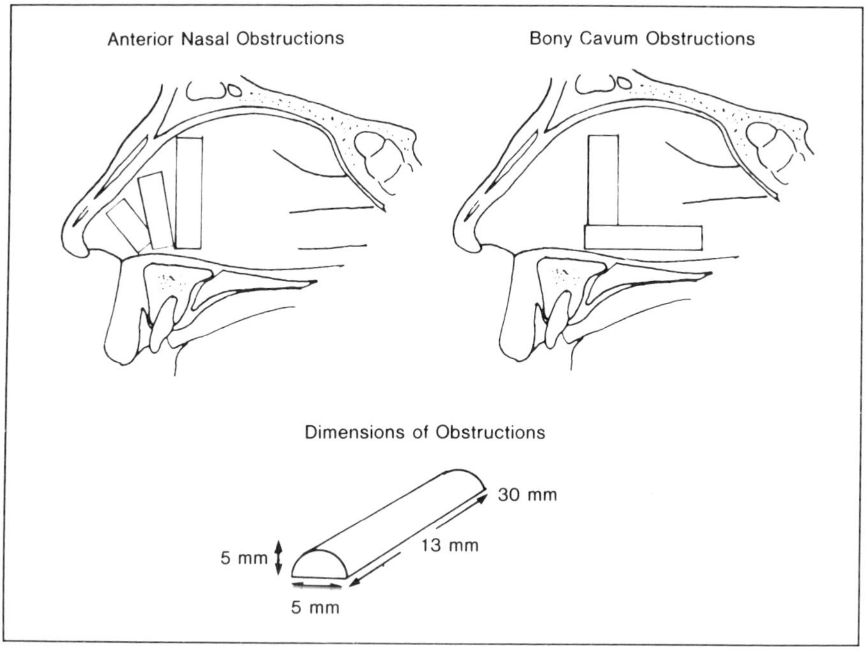

FIG 1–13.

Sites and sizes of simulated deviations. (From Chaban R, Cole P, Naito K: Simulated septal deviations (2). *Arch Otolaryngol Head Neck Surg* 1988; 114:413. Used by permission.)

Anterior Nasal Surgery

Surgery of the nasal tip and valve region demands superior judgment and precision[171, 172, 100] if risks of obstructive complications are to be avoided.[19, 20] Rhinomanometry has confirmed benefits of corrective septal surgery in this nasal segment,[124] and although it is widely accepted that corrective septal surgery with cartilage resection risks cosmetic defects from retraction of scar tissue, photographic studies before and 2 years after resection in patients whose dorsal and caudal cartilage struts had been preserved showed no cosmetic defect.[147]

Rhinomanometry has shown also that resistance to airflow is not necessarily increased by osteotomy and medial displacement of the nasal bones, even though this rhinoplastic procedure narrows the nose.[1, 15, 46] Moreover, the nasal valve is widened and stiffened by other rhinoplastic maneuvers such as "push-down"[6] and "rhinolift"[165] procedures. Nevertheless, cosmetic surgery is a common cause of alar obstruction,[22, 167] and many different procedures for relief of this unfortunate condition are described in

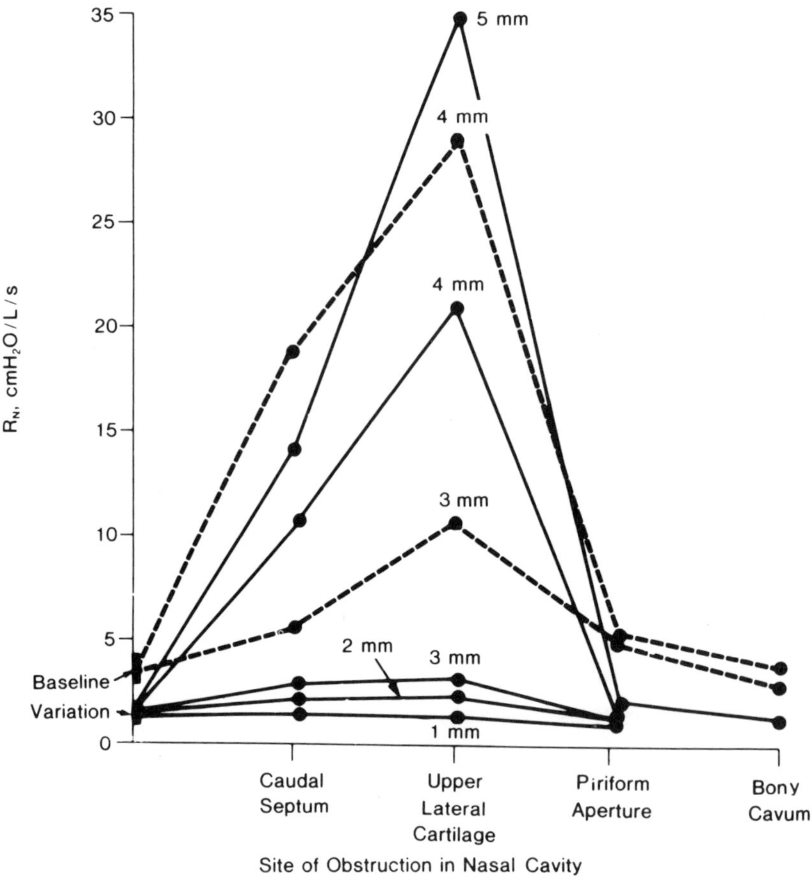

FIG 1–14.

Effect of thickness of simulated deviation on airflow resistance at different sites. Note marked differences between 3 and 4 mm at caudal septum and upper lateral cartilage sites. *Broken line* = decongested. (From Cole P, Chaban R, Naito K, et al: The obstructive nasal septum: Effect of simulated deviations on nasal airflow resistance. *Arch Otolaryngol Head Neck Surg* 1988; 114:410. Used by permission.)

the literature. Yet, objective postoperative assessments of the results are rarely reported.

Objective measurements have demonstrated that rapid maxillary expansion, a common orthodontic procedure (Fig 1–16), in addition to enlarging the upper dental arch, widens the piriform aperture and results in a marked and lasting increase in nasal patency.[189, 69, 183] This method has been employed as one of the alternatives in management of obstructive narrowing in the valve region.[177, 69]

Another procedure that is performed primarily for orthodontic or cosmetic purposes, LeFort 1 maxillary repositioning, also brings about an objective increase in nasal patency.[182]

Several different prosthetic devices are available for insertion into the vestibule to increase patency of the anterior nose and thus aid nasal breathing.[110, 145] But therapeutic use of these devices to relieve breathing disorders in sleep has been disappointing (see Chapter 2, "Snoring").

> **Clinical comment:** Minor structural or mucosal displacements of the medial and/or lateral walls of the nasal valve result in major changes in cross-sectional area and exponential changes in airflow resistances and transmural pressures.

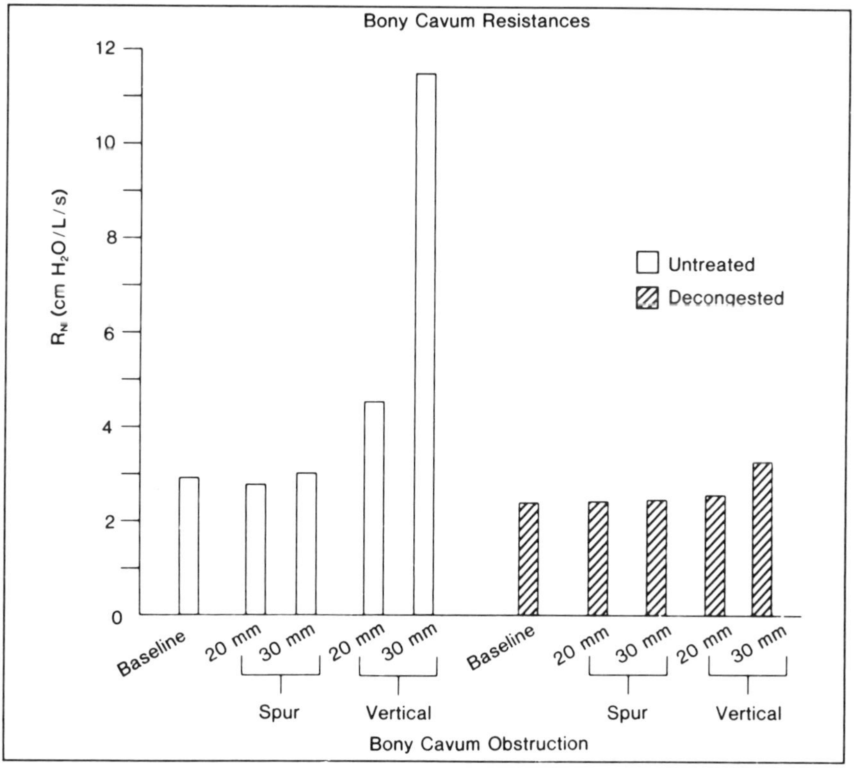

FIG 1–15.

Obstruction of caval lumen requires quite large simulated swelling. (From Chaban R, Cole P, Naito K: Simulated septal deviations (2). *Arch Otolaryngol Head Neck Surg* 1988; 114:413. Used by permission.)

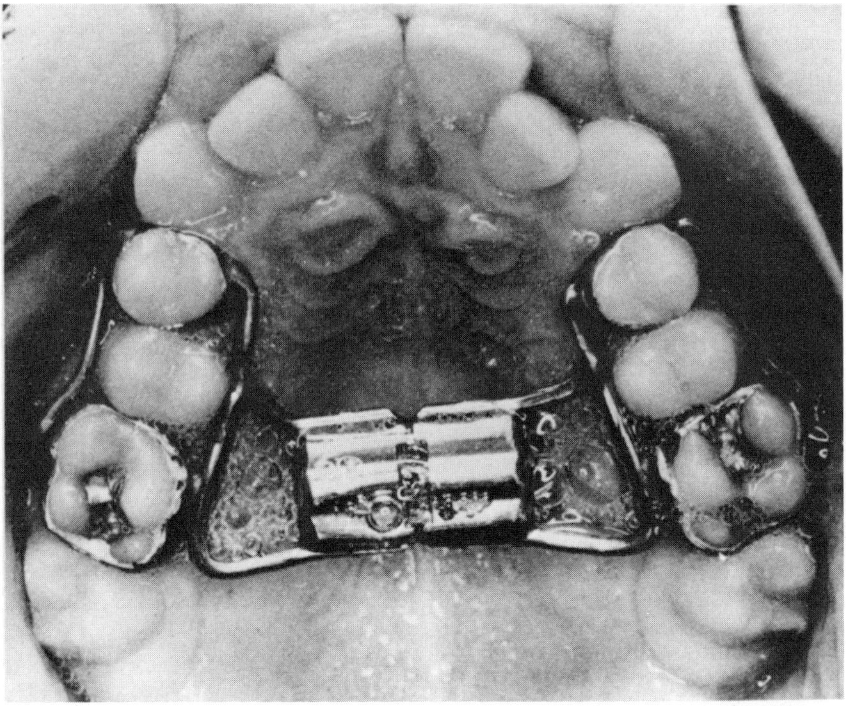

FIG 1–16.
Orthodontic device expanding palate by separation of midline suture. (From White BC, Woodside DG, Cole P: Effect of rapid maxillary expansion on nasal airway resistance. *J Otolaryngol* 1989; 18(4):137. Used by permission.)

ERECTILE MUCOSA

Resistive Effects

Mucosa, superimposed on structural elements of the stabilized anterior nose and the rigid bony cavum, narrows the skeletal nasal lumen; and at critical sites, notably the valve, airflow resistances are altered substantially by physiologic and pathologic changes in the degree of mucosal swelling (Poiseuille). This variable mucosal contribution to nasal airflow resistance is dependent mainly on the blood content of capacitance vessels that constitute the erectile components of the septal and lateral nasal walls (Figs 1–17 and 1–18).

Responses of these tissues to a variety of stimuli and emotional states[91] were recognized and demonstrated early in this century[179] by intra-

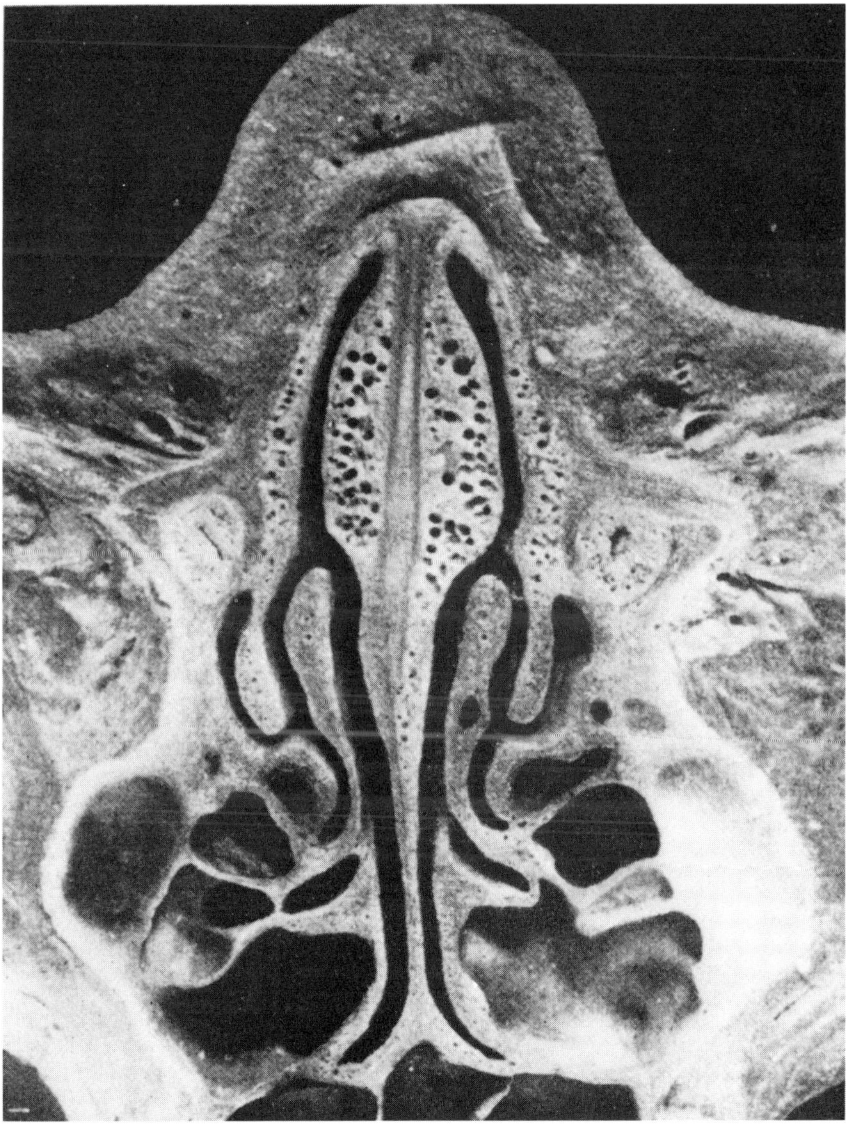

FIG 1–17.

Section of cadaver specimen of nasal cavity emphasizing capacitance vessels of erectile tissues dilated by injection material. Note septal body and vessels of the anterior lateral wall. (From Wustrow F: Schwellkorper am Septum nasi. *Z Anat Entwicklung* 1951; 116:139. Used by permission.)

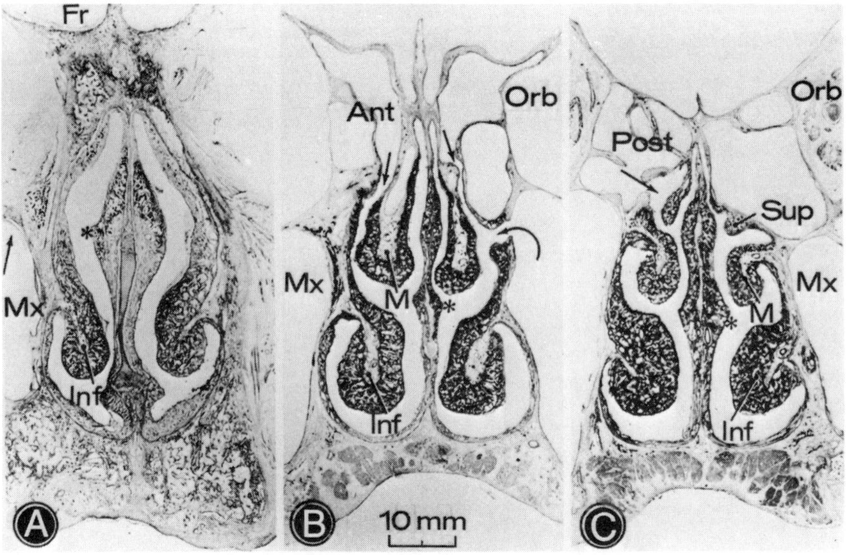

FIG 1–18.

Anterior **(A),** middle **(B),** and posterior **(C)** sections of nasal cavities demonstrating distribution of erectile tissues. (From Cauna N: Blood and nerve supply of the nasal lining, in Proctor DF, Anderson IB (eds): *The Nose: Upper Airway Physiology and the Atmospheric Environment.* Amsterdam, Elsevier Biomedical Press, 1982, p 46. Used by permission.)

nasal plethysmographic methods that are used by investigators to the present day.[57]

Nasal Capacitance Vessels

Nasal capacitance vessels respond appropriately to respiratory demands of exercise (Fig 1–19) and to several different local and remote stimuli (see following discussion) by constriction or by dilation, with corresponding adjustments of airway lumen. In many respects these vessels differ from capillaries and resistance vessels in their responses—for example, to vasoactive substances, to exercise, or to temperature.[144, 140, 115, 116, 121] They differ also in their function (Fig 1–20).

Nasal capacitance vessels regulate airway lumen and airflow resistance by changes in volume of their blood content: blood flow through them is of minor importance to this function. By contrast, nasal capillaries and resistance vessels, which include arteriovenous shunts, are concerned with metabolic and heat exchanges, and blood flow through them is adjusted to meet these requirements.[121, 138, 49, 82, 14] Blood flow through nasal mucosa of 30 ml/min/100 gm in the healthy young adult varies directly with inspiratory air temperature and inversely with age. It is increased in the presence of acute rhinitis and reduced in the allergic response.[13] Blood content and airflow resistance are both reduced by physical exercise, but blood flow is unchanged.[144]

Hypercapnia, hypoxia, and exercise bring about a constriction of nasal capacitance vessels that increases airway patency. Constriction is abolished by stellate ganglion or other sympathetic block.[152] Dilation takes place in

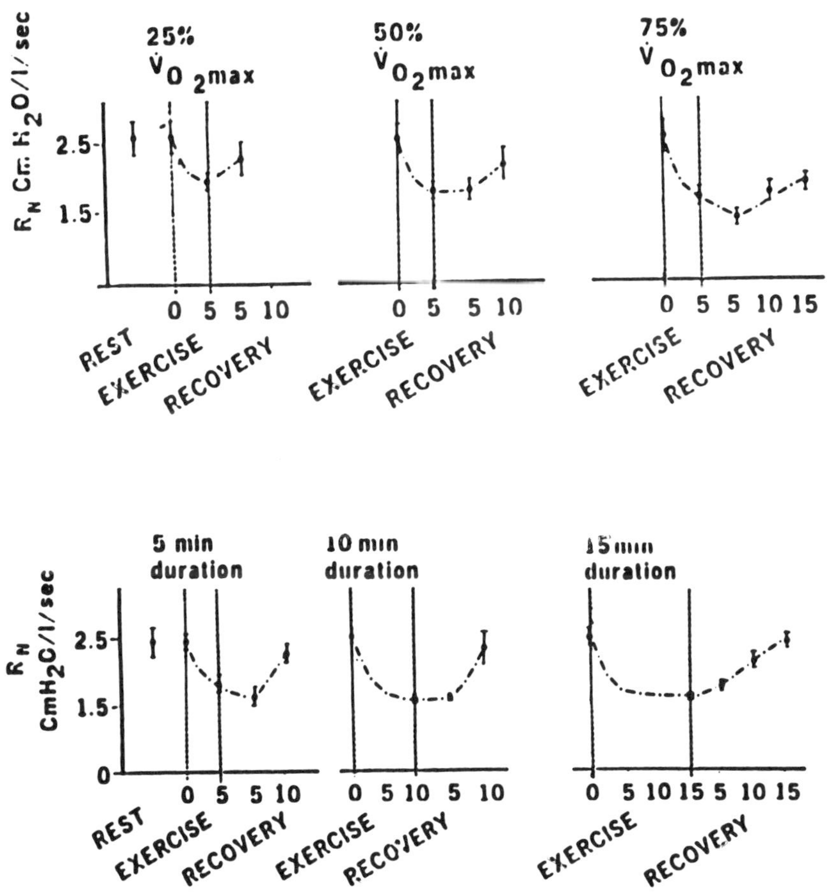

FIG 1–19.

Nasal resistive response to exercise and recovery. Note rapid and substantial decrease in resistance. Recovery requires 10 to 15 minutes. (From Forsyth RD, Cole P, Shephard RJ: Exercise and nasal patency. *J Appl Physiol* 1983; 55(3):860. Used by permission.)

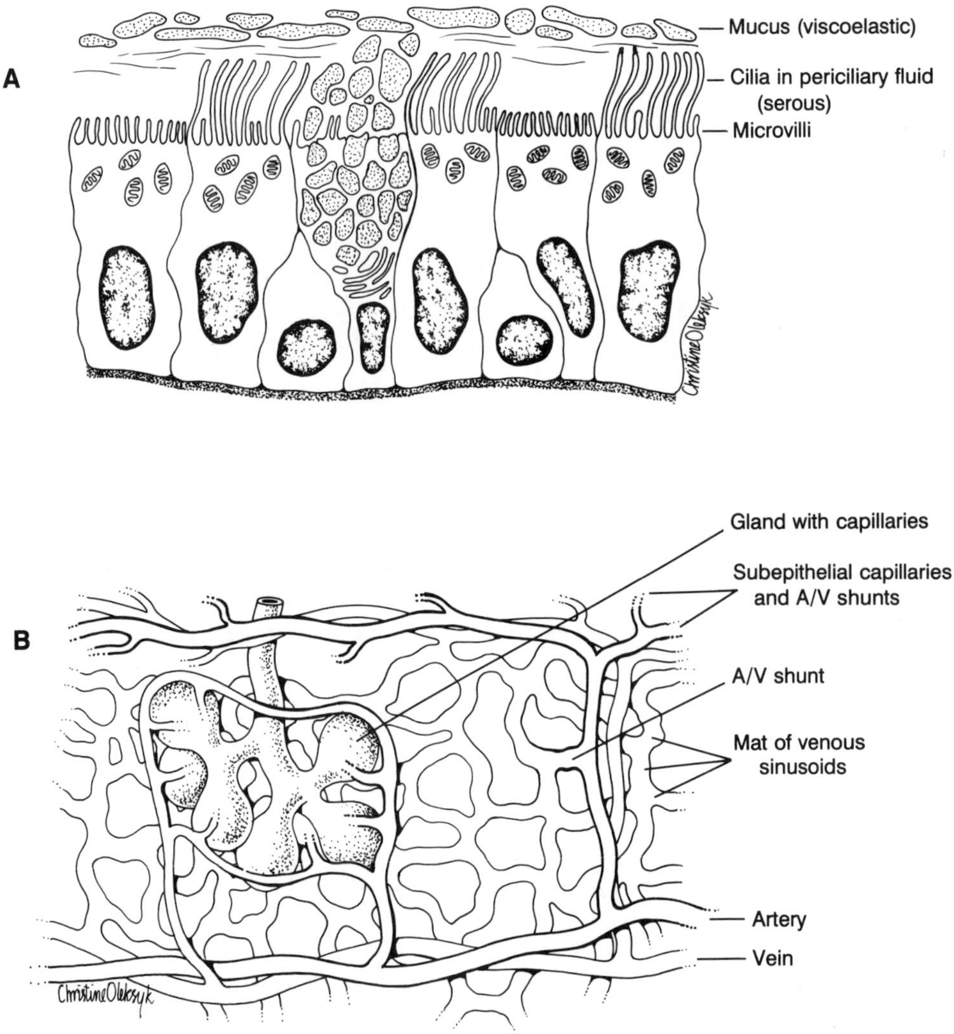

FIG 1–20.

Diagrammatic representation of sections of nasal mucosa emphasizing the major elements referred to in the text. **A,** epithelium, greatly magnified, **B,** subepithelial gland and vascular tissue, lesser magnification.

response to hyperventilation, nasal irritants, or cold inspiratory air.[48, 41, 123] Spontaneous and induced reciprocation of constriction and congestion between capacitance vessels of the separate nasal cavities is described later in this chapter.

Erectile Tissue

Erectile tissues are congested by the inflammatory process. Inflammation brings about a paresis of vascular tone[154, 155, 86] that allows capacitance vessels to fill with blood, and the airways may be narrowed further by accumulation of extravascular fluid and by the secretions and transudate that accompany the inflammatory process (discussed later under "Rhinitis and Turbinate Hypertrophy").

Cadaver studies[196] (see Fig 1–17) demonstrate that erectile tissues of the septum and lateral nasal wall achieve particular prominence in the anterior nose. Their blood content regulates airway lumen and airflow resistance principally in the narrowed valve segment (Poiseuille). Similar tissues have been noted in the choanal region[3] but in a single subject neither histamine nor decongestant affected airflow resistance when applied directly through a septal perforation (avoiding ipsilateral anterior erectile tissue) to the choanal mucosa. Furthermore, in these experiments, anterior erectile mucosa was unaffected by posterior application of vasoactive substances.[74]

Injected cadaver specimens show erectile tissue as a venous mat 1 to 5 mm thick[10] consisting of an accumulation of tortuous, irregular, intercommunicating, valveless venous sinuses. These thin-walled vessels with a rich sympathetic nerve supply[26] (see Fig 1–18) terminate in muscular throttle veins that possibly regulate venous drainage.

In vivo, computed tomographic (CT) studies by both X-ray and magnetic resonance imaging (MRI) (Figs 1–21 to 1–25) confirm the distribution and activities of nasal erectile tissues that are demonstrated by airflow studies[35, 39, 198] (see Chapter 3). The spontaneous nasal cycle, responses to vasoactive substances, and responses to postural stimuli have been clearly displayed by these imaging techniques.[35, 39, 198] In addition, the studies validate the clinical observation that nasal erectile tissues accommodate to structural irregularities (see Figs 1–21 to 1–25). They maintain a remarkably constant airway width of 2 to 3 mm in the more patent nasal cavum despite septal irregularities.

The ability to adapt so as to maintain an appropriate airway is not unlimited, since structural irregularities, depending on their size and site, can result in intermittent obstruction by cyclic or postural mucosal swelling at a narrowed site or more persistent obstruction when pathological mucosal

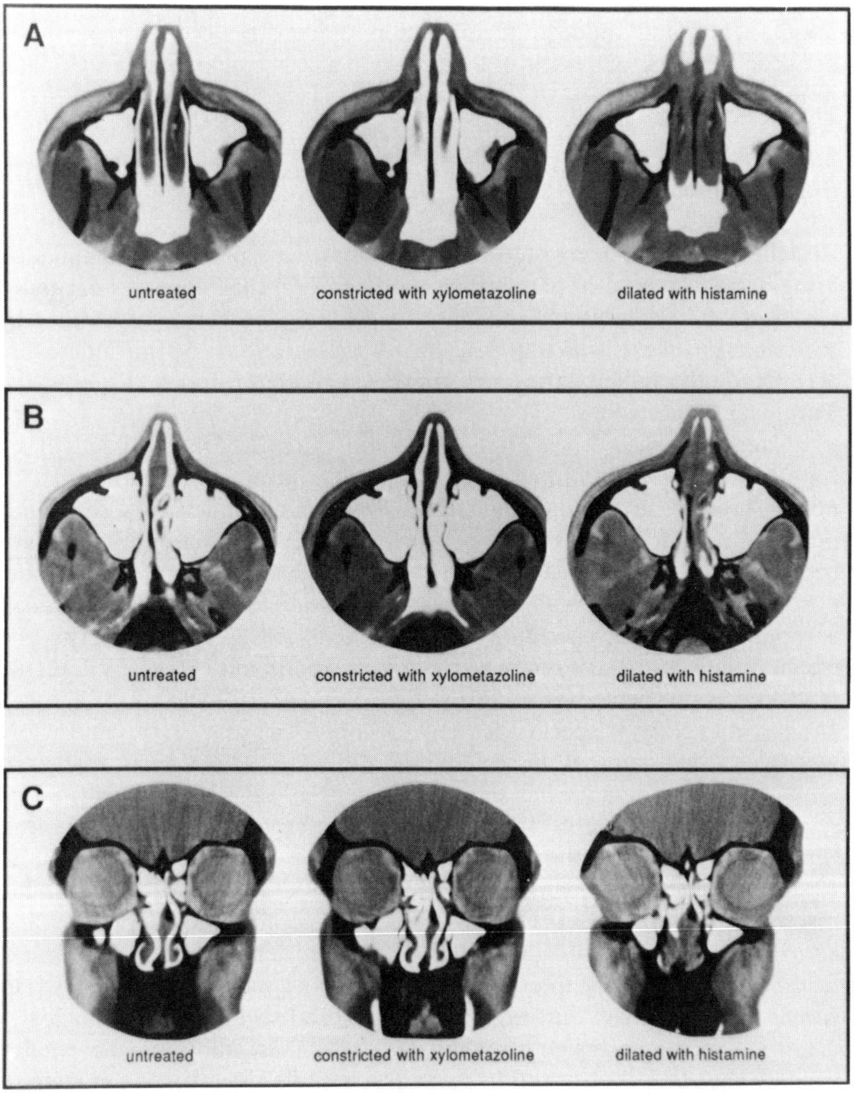

FIG 1–21.

Axial and coronal CT scans by X-ray. Responses of nasal erectile tissues to vasoactive substances. Note septal body and anterior projection of congested inferior turbinates. (From Cole P, Haight JSJ, Cooper PW, et al: A computed tomographic study of nasal mucosa: Effects of vasoactive substances. *J Otolaryngol* 1983; 12(1):58. Used by permission.)

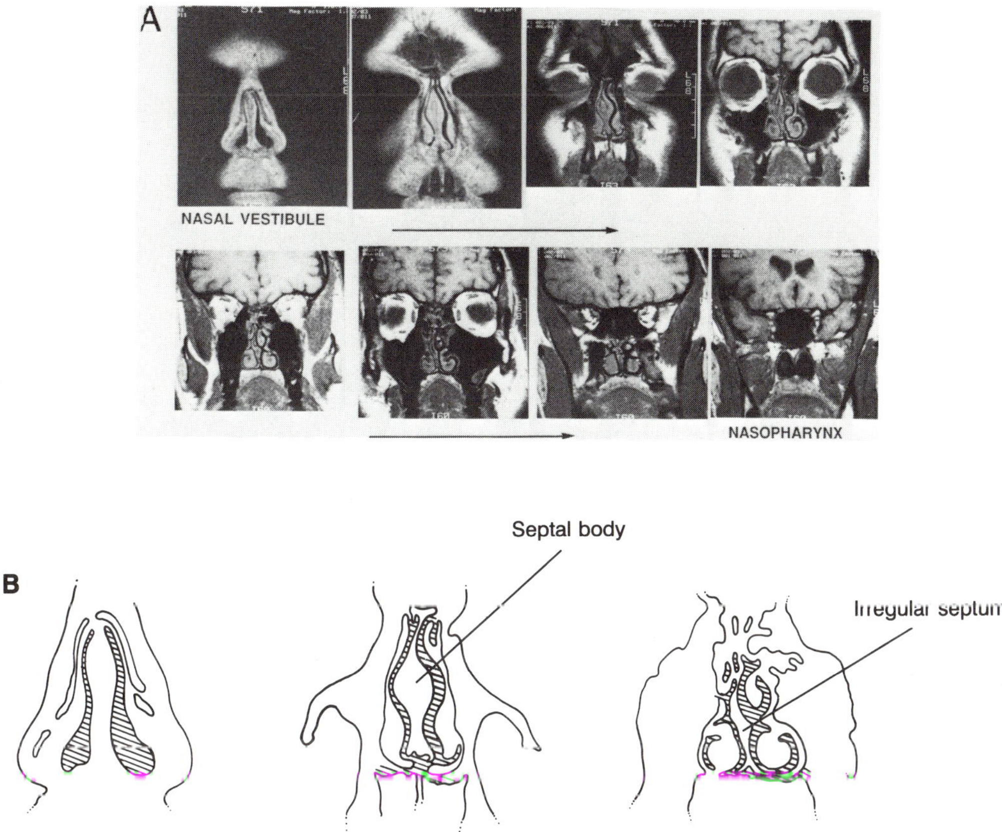

FIG 1–22.

Coronal MRI scans **(A)** and tracings **(B)** of nasal sections from vestibule to nasopharynx. Note obliquely sectioned valve region, anterior septal erectile body, and constant width of left airway despite septal irregularities. Asymmetry between airways is probably due to the phase of the cycle. (**A** from Cole P, Haight JSJ, Naito K, et al: Magnetic resonance imaging of the nasal airways. *Am J Rhinol* 1989; 3(2):63. Used by permission.)

swelling and/or skeletal deviation is severe. Resistive effects of structural irregularities or mucosal swelling are critical in the valve region, where the cross-sectional area is normally restricted (see Figs 1–3 to 1–6).[34]

Erectile tissue is not confined to the turbinates. In the congested nose, swelling of erectile tissue of the inferior turbinate is accompanied by swelling of the lateral nasal wall caudal (anterior) to it, and shrinking of these tissues with decongestant can be detected readily by rhinoscopy and demonstrated clearly by tomography (see Figs 1–21 to 1–25). These tissues of the lateral

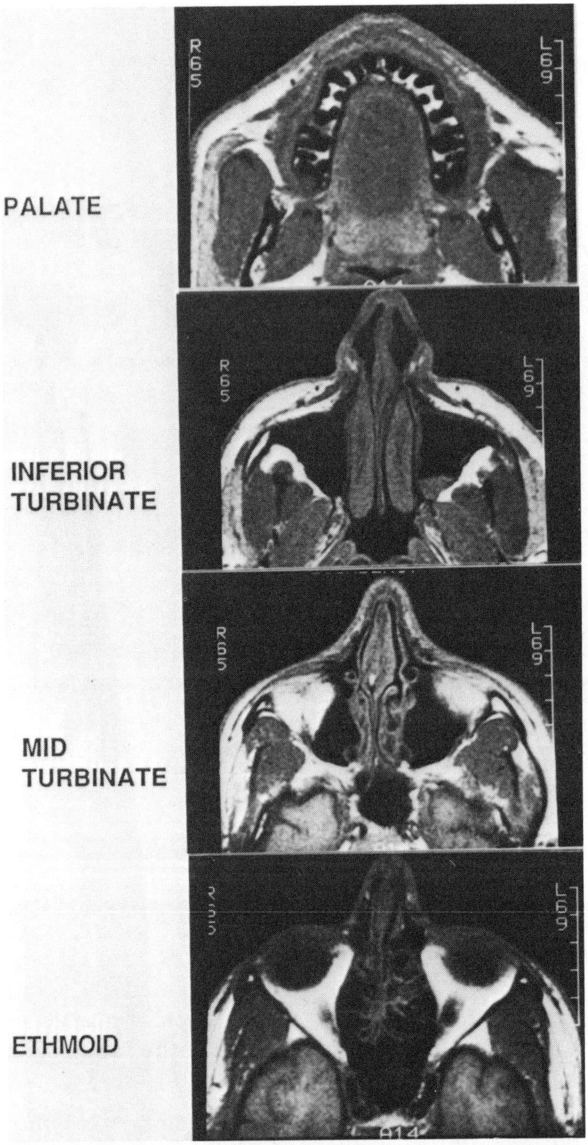

FIG 1–23.
Axial MRI scans. Note septal body anterior to middle turbinate and above inferior turbinate.

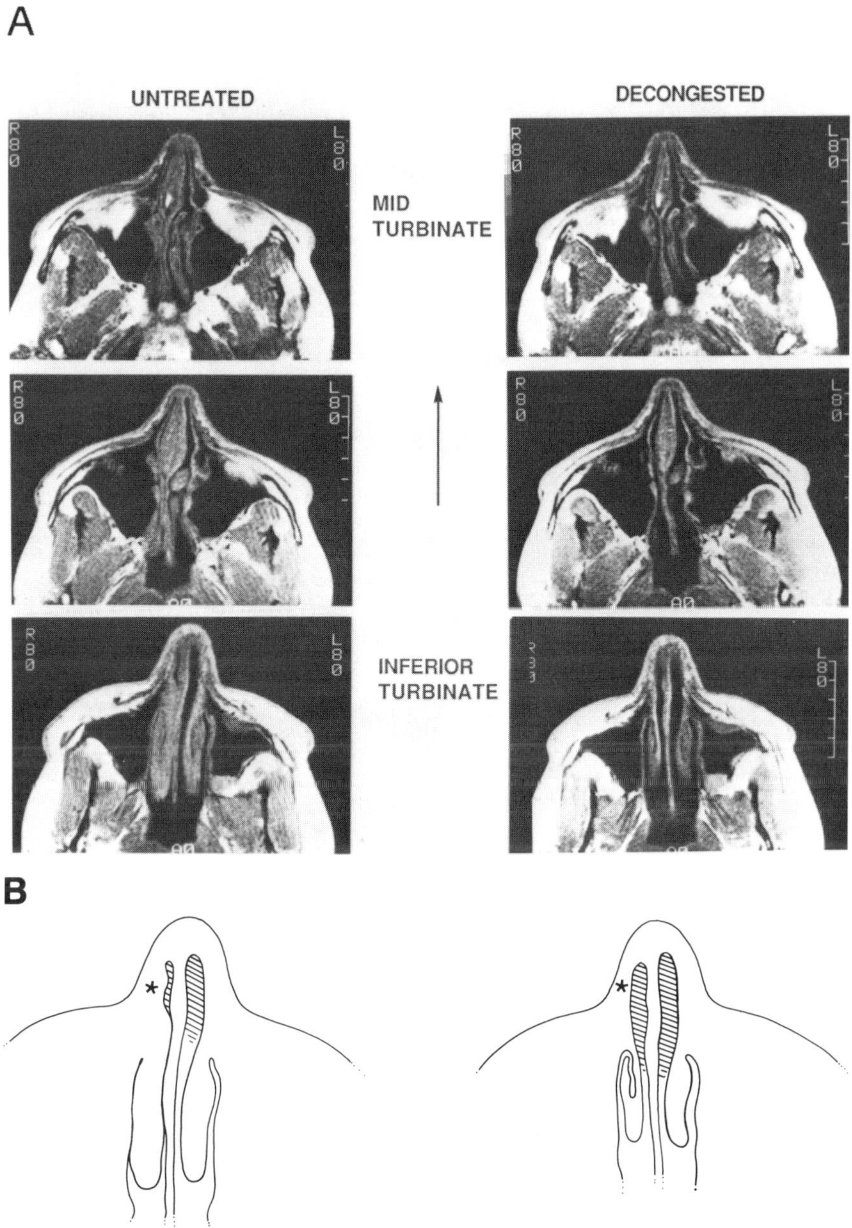

FIG 1–24.

Axial MRI scans **(A)** and tracings **(B).** Mucosa untreated and decongested. Note erectile tissue anterior to the inferior turbinate that shrinks with decongestant.

A

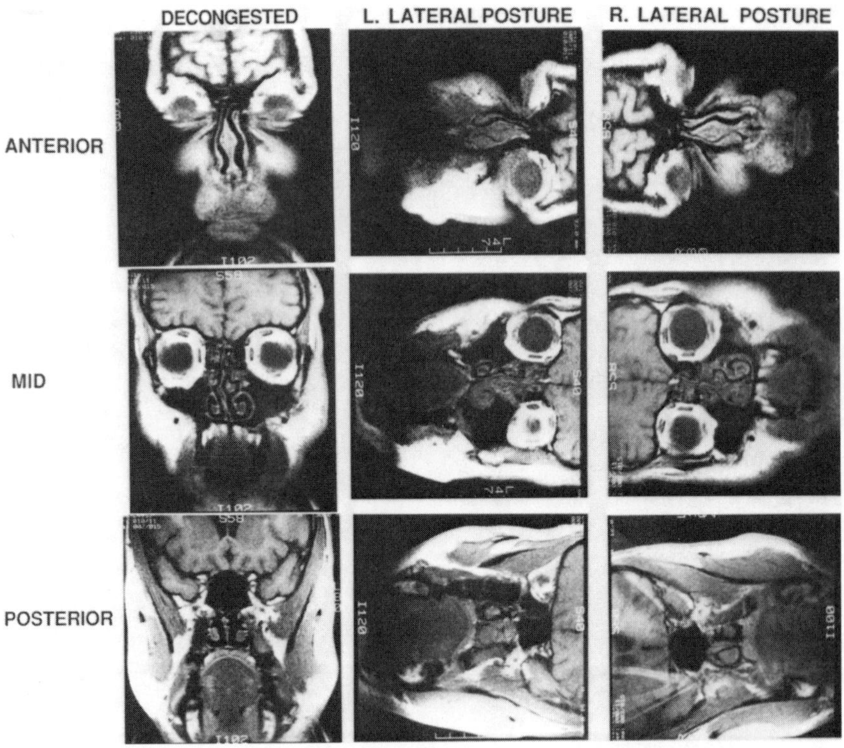

FIG 1–25.

Coronal MRI scans **(A)** and tracings **(B).** Effects of posture and decongestant. Note increased patency of the uppermost nasal cavity is of similar extent to that achieved by topical decongestant.

nasal wall that extend several millimeters beyond the piriform aperture when the mucosa is congested[94, 76] intrude on the lumen of the valve.

Substantial erectile tissues of the anterior septum, although clearly shown by cadaver and histologic studies and by tomographic studies in vivo, are less easy to gauge by rhinoscopy. The main mass of septal erectile tissue is located caudal (anterior) to the middle turbinate and dorsal (superior) to the inferior turbinate, but since these septal tissues are partially masked by the columella nasi, and the two sides cannot be viewed simultaneously, they are inconspicuous on rhinoscopic examination and are seldom direct targets of therapy (see the section on "Turbinectomy" in this chapter). However, elevation of the septal mucoperichondrium might inadvertently affect them in a way that contributes to the benefits of septoplasty.

B

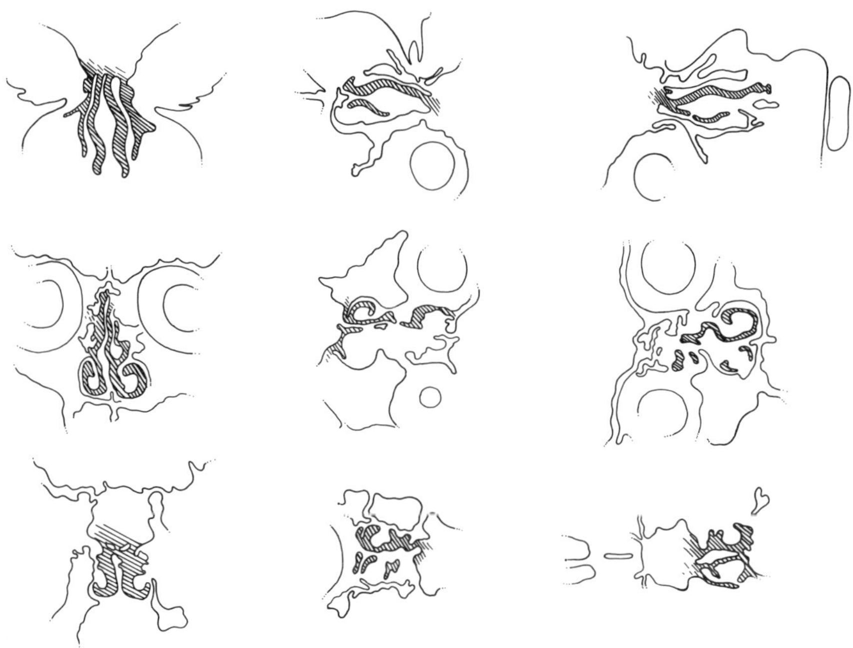

FIG 1-25 (cont.).
For legend, see opposite page.

> **Clinical comment:** Physiologic and pathologic changes in mucosal volume result predominantly from changes in blood content of capacitance vessels. Their effects on airflow resistance are critical at narrowed sites, principally in the anterior nose.

MUCOSAL DISEASE PREVALENCE

A Pervasive Disease

Population studies show a high incidence and prevalence of obstructive nasal mucosal diseases. Although obstructions of the hypopharynx, larynx, or trachea are much more dramatic and sometimes lethal, nasal obstructions rarely present acute threats to life, except possibly in infancy (see Chapter 2), since parallel nasal and oral passages provide alternative airways.

Yet nasal diseases seriously impair the quality of life and generate substantial economic consequences. Infective, acute and chronic, seasonal and perennial nasal diseases are commonplace and unpleasant not only to the sufferer, but also to others in the vicinity. Sniffling and a stuffy, running nose are socially distasteful, they are a source of embarrassment, and they provoke fears of infection in those around the sufferer. These diseases elicit little sympathy, medical treatment is often cursory, and in many cases the symptoms are reluctantly accepted as a miserable fact of life to be borne without hope of significant palliation.

These misery-producing nasal mucosal diseases result in diminished physical and mental performance and are responsible for absence from employment (more than 200 million workdays annually in the United States) and school. They account for extensive use of medical services and medications and pose a strong risk of complications, especially in the young, the aged, and the underprivileged. Adverse health effects result also from sleep fragmentation and from apneas that accompany inflammatory nasal obstruction since it is increased by recumbency (see Chapter 2).

Although even in developed countries, many patients do not seek professional help, nasal disorders account for approximately 15% of hospital ear, nose, and throat (ENT) outpatient attendance.[186] These diseases, along with associated upper respiratory ailments and their complications, occupy a major portion of the otolaryngologist's practice and are similarly demanding of the family practitioner,[185] the pediatrician, and the allergist.

In the course of a year, few people escape at least one attack of coryza, and some less fortunate suffer several attacks. Seasonal or perennial nasal allergies had a reported 1-year prevalence rate of 8% in a Michigan population study,[24] and as much as 21% seasonal and 5% perennial rhinitis has been reported among college students in Providence, Rhode Island.[161] It is estimated that more than 30 million US inhabitants suffer from hay fever (US National Center for Health Statistics). Similar figures have been cited in other Western countries[184] and less specific rhinitides increase these morbidity estimates substantially.

Toronto Studies

More than 20% of the population in developed countries suffers regularly from nasal obstruction. A 1987 questionnaire revealed that 34% of 719 randomly selected Toronto subjects aged 10 to 70 years were troubled by nasal symptoms.[23] Of 1,000 pediatric patients referred to the ENT Department at the Hospital for Sick Children, Toronto, with suspected nasal obstruction, elevated resistance was confirmed by rhinomanometry in 705. It was reduced substantially by topical decongestant in 410 patients in whom no structural nasal obstruction was detected, indicating mucosal disease with a major vascular component in almost two thirds of nasally obstructed pediatric patients. Adenoid enlargement, widely recognized as a cause of nasal obstruction in children, was diagnosed in approximately only one half the remainder.[143]

Lateral soft-tissue X-ray evaluation, a two-dimensional assessment of a three-dimensional situation,[54] confirmed the presence of enlarged adenoid in these patients, but adenoid and airway dimensions were poorly correlated with objective assessment of nasal airway patency.[47]

Sniffing and the Stuffy Nose

It has been suggested[25] that chronic sniffing and nasal obstruction maintain a vicious cycle and, indeed, erectile nasal mucosa is very labile in children[27] and inflamed mucosa is susceptible to engorgement by differential intranasal pressures[97] of a magnitude that can be readily attained by sniffing.

Upper and Lower Airway Diseases

The frequent coexistence of upper and lower respiratory airway diseases and reflex relationships between the upper and lower airways[190, 191, 197] reveal a unity of the respiratory tract,[40, 30] and findings of several workers suggest relationships between disordered nasal function and abnormalities in pulmonary function.[107, 137, 159, 194]

Clinical comment: Nasal obstruction afflicts "most of the people some of the time and some of the people most of the time." It results predominantly from impaired vascular tone and engorgement of capacitance vessels. It is exacerbated by structural irregularities and by recumbency.

RHINITIS AND TURBINATE HYPERTROPHY

Clinical Terminology

Clinicians use the terms *rhinitis* and *turbinate hypertrophy* rather indiscriminately. Rhinitis is not always inflammatory, and several nasal diseases, some clearly defined and others less so, come under its umbrella. Furthermore, obstructive turbinate swelling is usually vascular and occasionally edematous but seldom hypertrophic. "Hypertrophic" mucosal diseases are extremely common worldwide but, by contrast, atrophic rhinitis is rare in developed countries;[199] it accompanies cystic fibrosis,[112] and its reputation in association with turbinectomy is discussed in this chapter.

Classification

Rhinitis may be classified as infectious, seasonal allergic, perennial allergic, and perennial nonallergic. The latter category, usually diagnosed by exclusion, consists of eosinophilic and non-eosinophilic subgroups with the common synonym of vasomotor rhinitis. It is an allergy-like disease of unknown etiology;[131] indeed, histologic study of 1,500 nasal biopsies suggest it is not a single disease entity.[42] Autonomic imbalance as an explanation of this condition is unsubstantiated, and although vidian neurectomy is reported to control the paroxysmal rhinorrhea that afflicts older patients,[66] results of this procedure are less predictable in their effects on other manifestations of vasomotor rhinitis.

Nasal obstruction is a cardinal clinical feature of rhinitis. As already noted, not less than 20% of the population suffers regularly from it, and it is most common in young adults. Obstruction is frequently accompanied by discharge and not infrequently by sneezing and/or hyposmia. Rhinoscopy reveals characteristics of the mucosa and of the discharge helpful in diagnosis. Mucosal color reflects the status of superficial capillaries: red indicates dilation and brisk blood flow, a purplish tint suggests sluggish flow, and the pallor that is commonly seen in allergic states indicates constriction with little or no blood flow.[13] Turbinate swelling denotes congestion of the capacitance vessel system, and it may be augmented by extravascular fluid. Allergic discharge is typically clear and watery, viral infection produces a less specific mucoid discharge, and in cases of bacterial infection the discharge is purulent.

Infective Rhinitis

The nose is colonized by mixed bacteria. Many are pathogenic, and several possess the property of adherence to microvilli of nonciliated epithelial cells. Different bacteria are found predominantly, but not exclusively, at characteristic sites, such as *Staphylococcus pyogenes* in the vestibule and *Haemophilus influenzae, Streptococcus pyogenes,* and *Streptococcus pneumoniae* in the nasopharynx.

Viruses reside more briefly than bacteria; they exhibit marked antigenic heterogeneity and approximately 100 serotypes of rhinovirus have been identified. Some respiratory viruses proliferate most readily at temperatures $<37°$ C as are found in the nasal mucosa (see Chapter 3). It is of interest to note that traditional therapies for upper respiratory infections include warm blankets, a hot water bottle, and hot drinks—all measures that increase nasal mucosal blood flow and temperature (see Chapter 3, "Heat and Water Recovery"). Also "steam" inhalations that warm the mucosa are commonly employed, and therapeutic benefits of inhaling air saturated with water vapor at 42° to 44° C have been claimed.[141]

In addition to droplet transmission, bacteria and viruses can be transmitted to oral, nasal, or conjunctival membranes by contaminated fingers, since they can survive several hours on the skin (and other surfaces).

Mucosal Defenses

The mucociliary blanket furnishes the mucosa with several defenses in addition to a moving (6mm/min) mechanical barrier. Antibacterial and antiviral activity is provided by lactoferrin, lysozymes, and interferons contained in the low-viscosity periciliary fluid and the discontinuous visco-elastic clouds of mucus that are dragged along the serous surface by metachronous waves of the cilia tips (see Fig 1–20). Specific humoral immunity is afforded by secretion of both systemic and local IgA produced by plasma cells.[71] If these barriers against invasion are breached by desiccation, a virus, or a toxic substance, mucociliary function is disrupted and the mucosa becomes vulnerable to bacterial infection that produces further injury. Massive destruction of cilia occurs in the early days of rhinoviral infection, and recovery of functioning ciliated epithelium following acute injury requires as long as several weeks.[161] It may be incomplete months after *Mycoplasma* infection.

The relative nasal mucosal ischemia that accompanies chilling of the body[33, 55, 151] (see the summary in chapter 2) has been suggested as a predisposing factor in nasal infection. However, experiments in which human volunteers were wet and chilled following nasal innoculation with virus did not add strong support to this view.

Inflammatory Responses

The degree of inflammatory obstructive mucosal swelling reflects the blood content of the extensive system of capacitance vessels. Vascular tone is diminished by the inflammatory process, but the dilated capacitance vessels constrict with alacrity in response to an α-agonist or to vigorous exercise.[152] It seems that in most cases of nasal inflammatory disease the obstructive swelling and rapid decongestion are predominantly vascular phenomena[152] (see Fig 1–19). It is unlikely that a substantial extravascular-fluid component of the swelling would be so rapidly absorbed by lymphatic channels and by capillaries constricted in response to a decongestant.

Allergic and inflammatory nasal mucosal responses are accompanied by an accumulation of several vasoactive and secretomotor biochemical mediators derived in large part from mast-cell granules. They act directly on blood vessels and glands of the mucosa (Table 1–2). Their effects are modified by central, antidromic, and axonal nervous reflexes associated with several vasoactive neurotransmitters, in addition to acetylcholine and noradrenaline. Numerous neuropeptides (see Table 1–2) related with nonmyelinated trigeminal nerve fibers have been identified,[60, 192, 191] but in many cases their precise functions are unknown. No differentiated neural end-organs have been detected, and the naked terminations of peptidergic fibers that are present between epithelial cells and deep to them do not perforate tight epithelial junctions to reach the mucosal surface. In addition to their central sensory responses to touch, temperature, and irritants, these trigeminal nerve fibers serve vasomotor and secretomotor antidromic reflex functions.

TABLE 1–2.
Biochemical Mediators and Neuropeptides in Nasal Mucosal Responses

Mast Cell Mediators	Neuropeptides
Histamine	Calcitonin gene–related peptide
Bradikinin	Somatostatin
Leukotrienes	Substance P
Prostaglandins	Vasoactive intestinal peptide
Serotonin	Galanin
Chemotaxins	Neurokinins
Heparin	Gastrin releasing peptide
Trypsin	Neuropeptide Y
Adenosine	Peptide histidine isoleucine

Inflammatory rhinorrhea consists of increased serous and mucinous secretions augmented by desquamated epithelial cells, passage of cells and macromolecules through loosened junctions between epithelial cells, and an exudate of water, smaller molecules, and ions.[106, 193]

Allergic Responses

In the allergic state, basophils and mast cells originating from bone marrow proliferate and migrate within the nasal tissues and to the seromucinous fluid lining the nasal lumen.[128] Antigen dissolved from inhaled allergenic particles reacts with antigen-specific IgE attached to receptors on the surface of these cells and brings about the release of histamine and other mediators, resulting in an "immediate" inflammatory response (within minutes). In many cases it is followed after several hours by histamine release, an influx of neutrophils, macrophages, and eosinophils, and an accumulation of a variety of mediators, some of them cytotoxic. Basophils may play a greater role than mast cells in this delayed response.[29]

The return of mediators and of "late" symptoms can be inhibited by steroid, but antihistamine is effective only in blocking H_1 receptors, and other specific antimediator medications are not yet available.

Immediate and late responses prime the mucosa to react to nonspecific stimuli; this is a transient hypersensitivity that persists for several days and, together with a late type of reaction, may be responsible for chronicity of symptoms. It, too, is inhibited by steroid.[132] Nasal washings have shown topical steroid to reduce both cellular and humoral immediate and late responses in challenge experiments. Mediator release similar to the allergic response is brought about also by infecting bacteria and their products.

Eosinophil leucocytes are characteristically included in the allergic cellular response, but the nose is too small a shock organ to generate a marked increase in blood eosinophilia. These cells are stimulated by mediators, and they release substances toxic both to parasites and to respiratory epithelium. In addition to their presence in allergic disease nasal eosinophilic cells are found in many cases of nonallergic rhinitis.

Diagnosis and Treatment of Nasal Allergy

A confident diagnosis of nasal allergy can usually be made on the basis of patient and family history (the latter is positive in two thirds of cases) and clinical examination and skin testing (in vitro tests such as RAST are seldom required except for research purposes). It is axiomatic that the significance of skin tests be assessed in conjunction with other findings and that treatment be based on examination of the patient rather than on test results that can be noncontributory or even misleading.

Neonatal exposure that increases the risk of seasonal allergy many years later might be avoided by birth-date control by allergic parents. Indeed, avoidance of exposure to allergens is a primary preventive and therapeutic measure for susceptible subjects of all ages. If avoidance fails to alleviate allergic symptoms, systemic antihistamine H_1 inhibitors are useful in reducing sneezing, itching, rhinorrhea, and conjunctival symptoms. These medications are more effective in control of the immediate than the late phase reaction, as is also the prophylactic and frequent daily use of topical disodium cromoglycate, a mast-cell stabilizer,[119] but a topical or systemic decongestant is required to relieve established nasal congestion. A nonsedating H_1 inhibitor is a common first choice in the treatment of nasal allergy and the more recently developed members of this group of medications, in addition to a diminished central nervous sedative effect, may exert a wider impact than H_1 receptor blockade.[99]

As an effective alternative to antihistamine, steroid therapy, either systemic or topical, controls nasal allergic symptoms in the majority of patients.[160] Systemic treatment is reserved for refractory cases or for the initiation of topical steroid therapy in particularly severe cases. Application of any one of the topical steroids that have been developed for control of nasal allergic symptoms is effective in the majority of afflicted patients, and these medications offer an additional and important advantage over antihistamines in reducing mucosal swelling. Topical steroid provides effective treatment also in many cases of nonallergic rhinitis, notably those with nasal eosinophilia.[127]

Patients should be warned that the instant relief of a topical decongestant is not to be expected with this therapy, and several days of maximal recommended dosage of topical steroid may be required before a symptomatic response is noticeable. When symptomatic control is established, minimal steroid dosage can then be determined by trial and error and continued as long as necessary to maintain control. The frequency of topical application can be successfully reduced to less than daily in some cases. Synergism between antihistamine and steroid may enable dosage of each to be minimized.[99]

Topical Steroid

Topical steroid medications in therapeutic dosage have been used extensively for many years and for lengthy periods of treatment without serious local or systemic side effects. Rarely septal perforations have been reported,[160] but whether they result from mode of application, the propellant, the steroid, or from an unrelated cause is unclear. To avoid this possibility, application should not be directed against the septum.

Scanning electron microscopy has shown no recognizable mucosal abnormalities following 12 months' continuous use of topical beclomethasone[130] and the small quantities of steroid that are absorbed into the circulation by passage through the nasal mucosa (15%) and by swallowing and ingestion are rapidly removed from the bloodstream. They are rendered inactive by a single pass through the liver and do not disturb endogenous steroid metabolism in dosage recommended by the manufacturer. The half-life of the more recently developed topical steroids after absorption and distribution throughout the body tissues is <3 hours.

Immunotherapy

Immunotherapy by specific desensitization is a therapeutic measure widely recommended by allergists.[127] Immune responses of increased IgG blocking antibody and reduction of antibody specific IgE to this form of therapy have been demonstrated,[120] and some patients show a favorable clinical response by reduction of symptoms and/or requirements for medication.[64] There is evidence also that immunotherapy for nasal allergy can reduce the risk of subsequent development of asthma.[120] Sixty percent of asthmatic patients suffer from allergic rhinitis, and 20% of patients with allergic rhinitis are asthmatic.[161] Specific desensitization requires a lengthy period of injections, which undoubtedly help some patients suffering from seasonal allergies, but results are unpredictable in the individual case and many of the failures turn to the otolaryngologist for further help.

Clinical comment: Inflammatory nasal mucosal disease is widespread globally. Of the many medications available for treatment of the pervasive noninfective rhinitides, topical steroid is safe, effective, and a first choice of many practitioners. Antihistamines, preferably nonsedating, cromolyn sodium, and specific desensitization are alternatives.

TURBINECTOMY

Atrophic Rhinitis

The risk of atrophic rhinitis following turbinectomy has been emphasized in rhinological teaching for much of this century. Yet, clinical experience and an increasing number of publications cast doubt on the inevitability of this disastrous consequence. Although it is reported[126] (and denied[142]) that total turbinectomy is accompanied by significant morbidity, it does not appear to be a serious consequence of several injurious and widely employed treatments of the inferior turbinates. These treatments include crushing, fracturing, partial excision, submucosal resection, topical cautery by chemicals or diathermy, submucosal sclerosants or diathermy, thermocautery, cryosurgery and even vaporization by laser.

Cases of atrophic rhinitis following these widely practiced procedures have not been reported in the literature, and the cases of atrophic rhinitis that have been reported did not follow turbinate surgery.[45]

The disease of atrophic rhinitis is rare in developed countries;[199] and even in dry, dusty, tropical Nigeria,[135] where a long-term study was undertaken, it has been reported that total turbinectomy provided effective relief of obstructive nasal symptoms and did not result in atrophic rhinitis. Most complications of turbinate reduction that have been reported appear minor or avoidable.[50] Although one would not advocate destructive measures lightly, it seems that risks of atrophy may be exaggerated.[1]

Diathermy and Cryosurgery

Both rhinomanometry and symptomatology show increased nasal patency 2 months after submucosal diathermy in humans.[96] Animal studies[103] have demonstrated complete healing and reduced mucosal thickness after a similar period following cryosurgery. It is of interest also that although biopsies taken 6 weeks after diathermic turbinate treatment have shown fibrosis and reduction of vascular tissue,[96] histology of biopsy specimens taken before and several months after these destructive procedures exhibit no distinguishing differences of scar tissue or vascularity.[78] It appears that scarring is temporary and that capacitance vessels can regenerate.

Interpretation of results of turbinate reduction is frequently complicated by its combination with other procedures for increasing nasal patency. There are few conclusive studies allowing comparisons of effectiveness among the many different turbinate therapies. It seems probable that diathermy can provide considerable temporary relief,[95, 93] but postoperative assessment at 2 years shows little permanent benefit.[78]

Reduction Turboplasty

Anterior reduction turboplasty is widely practiced for obstructive turbinate enlargement, and both rhinomanometry[195, 166] and acoustic rhinometry[113] (see Fig 4–1) have demonstrated that increased nasal patency results. Although there is little difference in the short-term between anterior and total inferior turbinectomy as regards the reduction of nasal airflow resistance, patients experience a greater sensation of patency following the more radical procedure, and the results of that procedure appear more durable.[195] It should be noted also that a series of results has been reported that demonstrates little difference in nasal resistances following anterior and posterior turbinectomy.[178]

Extraturbinate Erectile Tissues

In addition to the turbinates, extensive erectile tissues of the anterior septum have been demonstrated, and lack of specific surgical attention to both medial and lateral nasal erectile tissues, especially those situated anteriorly, might account for some of the failures of turbinate treatment[78] (see Figs 1–21 to 1–25). Indeed, residual or recurrent erectile tissue has been noted on the anterior lateral nasal wall in cases of unsuccessful relief of obstruction by turbinectomy,[195] and substantial erectile tissues anterior to the inferior turbinate bone can be seen clearly in histologic and tomographic sections of normal noses (see "Erectile Mucosa" earlier in this chapter). The importance of erectile tissues in the anterior nose to airflow resistance is highlighted by the negligible change in nasal patency that has been reported to follow excision of the entire lateral wall of the cavum of patients in the course of tumor surgery.[133]

It has been suggested that benefits of turbinate surgery might be due not only to reduction of tissue volume but also to nerve destruction and resulting altered sensation or, alternatively, to diminution of neurogenic sensitivity and reduction of hyperactivity.

Clinical comment: Destruction of chronically swollen nasal erectile tissue effectively increases patency in cases of failed medical treatment. Of the many methods, judicious excision appears the most effective and durable. Fears of atrophic rhinitis are exaggerated. Residual erectile tissue may account for some surgical failures.

THE NASAL CYCLE

A Biological Rhythm?

In health, alternations of nasal congestion and decongestion are manifested as a resistive cycle, but healthy subjects are usually unaware of these shifting resistances—even though they can fluctuate unilaterally between severe obstruction and optimum patency (Fig 1–26). The absence of sensation of airway resistance and patency might be explained partially by cyclical reciprocity between sides that minimizes alteration of combined resistances of the paired nasal cavities.[168, 169] However, this resistive homeostasis can be disturbed by structural asymmetry of the nasal cavities or by inflammatory mucosal diseases and thus result in obstructive symptoms[7, 136, 31] (Fig 1–27).

The apparently spontaneous[72] nasal cycle is irregular in frequency and amplitude,[43] and minor fluctuations of brief duration are superimposed upon its leisurely progression, but reciprocity between sides is fairly consistent.[90, 75, 98] Although the phenomenon may not satisfy all criteria of

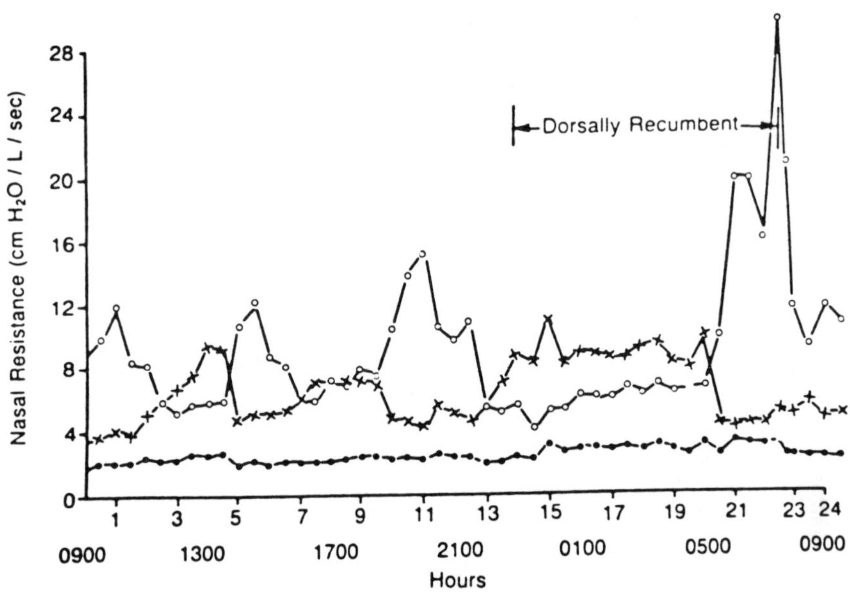

FIG 1–26.
Nasal cycle recorded over a 24-hour period in a healthy adult subject. Note reciprocation of resistances between left *(crosses)* and right *(open circles)* sides and stability of combined resistances *(closed circles)*. (From Cole P, Haight JSJ: Posture and the nasal cycle. *Ann Otol Rhinol Laryngol* 1986; 95:233. Used by permission.)

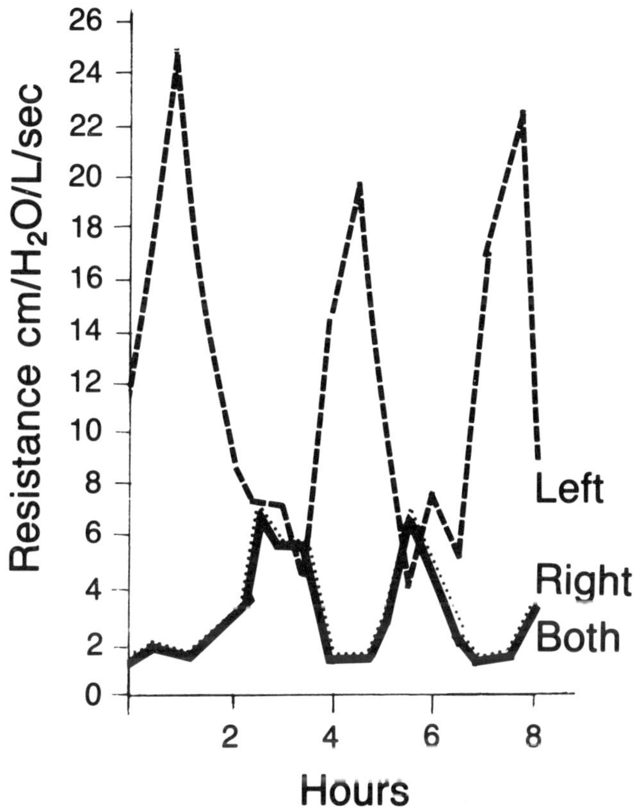

FIG 1–27.

Nasal cycle in patient with obstructive left septal deviation. Note that reciprocation exists, but the structurally more patent nasal cavity *(right)* is the main determinant of combined nasal resistances that fluctuate with the cycle. Contrast with Fig 1–26 in which combined resistances *(solid line)* do not fluctuate with cycle. (From Cole P: Stability of nasal airflow resistance. *Clin Otolaryngology Allied Sci* 1989; 14:177–182. Used by permission.)

cyclical activity and may be episodic rather than periodic,[65] the term *nasal cycle* is well established and widely recognized.

This curious cycle was first described in Western rhinology almost a century ago.[102] It has been recognized in Yogic literature for several centuries[164] and is regarded as a sign of good health. Furthermore, modification of the cyclical phases by pressures exerted in the axillary region (see later discussion) and by breathing maneuvers plays an important role in pranayama yoga breathing exercises.[18, 181, 162, 163]

Characteristics of the Nasal Cycle

The nasal cycle can be demonstrated in most adults[104, 88] and in children and infants.[109] Ipsilaterally increased secretion is reported to accompany each decongestive phase.[114] A similar resistive cycle has been demonstrated in several mammals, including cats, dogs, pigs, rabbits and rats. These animals exhibit erectile tissue in and around the internal nasal ostium.[56, 17]

The cycle is present in sleeping humans.[92] It is unaffected by topical anesthesia or acute nasal occlusion[104] but is suppressed by tracheostomal breathing, and it returns on resumption of use of the natural airway.[87] It is abolished temporarily by topical decongestant and, if the decongestant is applied unilaterally, the cycle continues contralaterally.[149] Since the cycle and several resistive responses to different stimuli are abolished by decongestant and yet are manifested when the alae are immobilized by splinting, they are clearly vascular manifestations and not the result of alar activity.

Other Synchronous Cycles

Other cyclical phenomena showing lateralization synchronous with the nasal cycle have been reported in humans. They include electrocortical activity,[188, 187] sweating,[111] pupil size, conjunctival capillary diameter,[11] and even cognitive performance.[105] Moreover, as described below, unilateral nasal decongestion results also from contralateral pressures applied to the body surface, and it is accompanied by ipsilateral congestion.[77, 75, 73, 79, 80] Sweat secretion also responds contralaterally to posture and body-surface pressures,[108, 59, 175, 101, 174] and both nasal and sweat responses appear to be mediated by a similar sympathetic route.

The preceding observations suggest that the nasal cycle and its modifications are sensitive indicators of widely distributed reciprocating neuro-autonomic activity; and although they provide an interesting source of speculation, these vascular responses do not necessarily perform a functionally useful role in the nose.

Posture and Pressure Effects

The cycle is overridden by reciprocal vascular responses of the nasal mucosa to lateral recumbent postures[36] and to pressures applied unilaterally to the body surface even in the upright subject[37, 73, 79, 80] (Fig 1–28). Under these conditions, in which contralateral decongestion and ipsilateral congestion

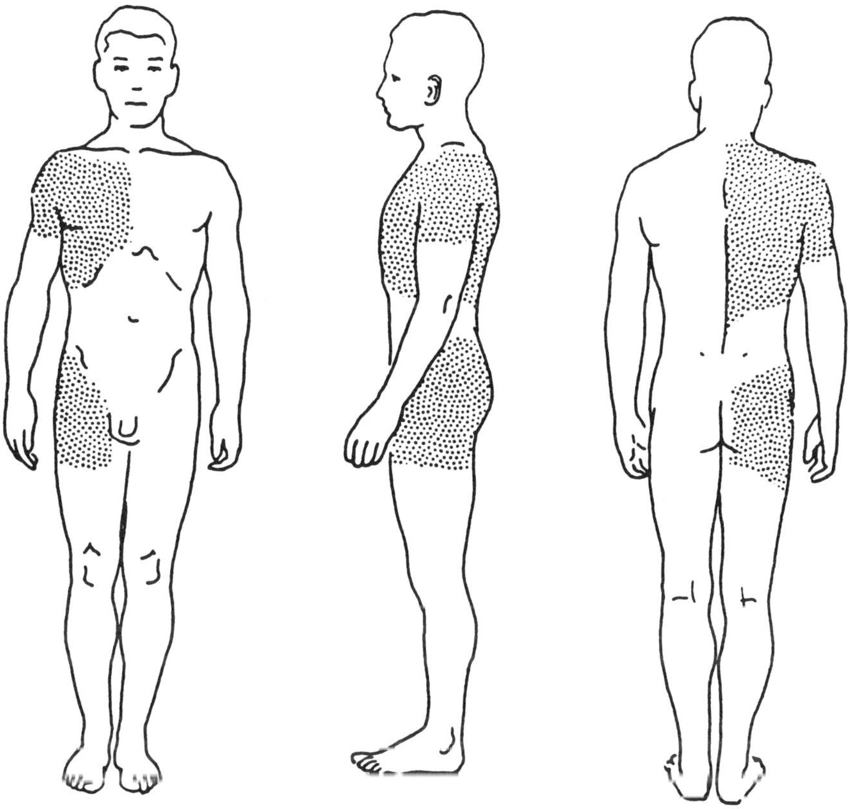

FIG 1–28.

Body surfaces from which pressures elicit contralateral nasal decongestion and homolateral congestion. (From Haight JSJ, Cole P: Topographical anatomy of the pressure points that alter nasal resistance. *J Otolaryngol* 1986; 15(suppl 16):14. Used by permission.)

are induced by the stimulus, reciprocity continues to minimize change in airflow resistance of the combined nasal cavities.

The nasal response that accompanies lateral chest-wall pressure takes place despite local anesthesia of the skin but could not be elicited following intercostal nerve block in a single subject who was otherwise consistently responsive.[73, 79, 80] It seems that the receptors involved in the reflex are deeply situated, and it is of interest to note that the nasal reflex responses are not elicited by unilateral superficial thermal or painful stimuli.

The cycle is reset by the assumption of a lateral recumbent posture, the upper side becoming more patent and the lower more resistive. Periodic reciprocation begins anew if this lateral posture is maintained for a sufficiently lengthy period, but resistive responses are temporary and progression of the cycle does not appear to be affected by brief periods of lateral recumbency.[73, 79, 80]

In standing subjects, amplitude of the cycle is much smaller than in seated or recumbent subjects,[36] and nasal resistances are unaffected by weight-bearing on one foot or the other. Absence of stimuli from gravitational pressures on the body surface or action of the cardiovascular homeostatic reflex of capacitance vessels[153] might account for the amplitude differences.

There is no great change in total resistance of the combined nasal cavities of the healthy nose as a subject alters position from seated to dorsal recumbency.[85, 155] The cyclically decongested side is little affected, and the congested side, where vascular tone is reduced, responds to hydrostatic change by further dilation of capacitance vessels, thus increasing its already high resistance. Nevertheless, although severe unilateral obstruction has been noted in recumbent and sleeping subjects, increases in resistance of the congested nasal cavity do not exert a major effect on total nasal resistance.[92]

In the inflamed nose, where vascular tone is decreased on each side, the total nose becomes congested and increasingly obstructed on assumption of a dorsal recumbent posture.[86, 154] In the upright posture, the cycle is modified by structural (see Fig 1–27) or mucosal nasal diseases, and stabilizing reciprocal adjustments are disrupted.[136]

Clinical comment: Spontaneous and induced congestive vascular changes of the nasal mucosa are ceaseless and frequently reciprocal; they entail flow-resistive, symptomatic, and rhinoscopic consequences.

DECONGESTION

A Vascular Phenomenon

Nasal epithelial cells whose surface areas are increased enormously by 300 to 400 microvilli, like those in the gut, can transport water-soluble substances applied to their surfaces rapidly to subepithelial tissues, capillaries,[26] and capacitance vessels. The nasal vascular response to topical application of an α-agonist decongestant in therapeutic concentration usually results in a marked increase in nasal patency within a few moments. This rapid nasal route to the circulation is therefore employed also for the administration of different medications[150] and other substances[63] in addition to those used in the treatment of nasal disease (e.g., antidiuretic hormone).

The degree of decongestion is dose-dependent[12] and xylometazoline, an α_1-agonist, reduces both nasal mucosal blood flow and blood content while phenylephrine, an α_2-agonist reduces only blood content.[4] Differences in vascular behavior as between capacitance and resistance vessels,[115, 49] are found also between capillaries (open diameter 5 to 10 μm) and the muscular arteriovenous shunts (open diameter 150 μm) as, for instance, to sympathetic stimulation.[5]

Topical decongestant or congestant (e.g., histamine) applied unilaterally to the human nose has been found not to affect contralateral patency during quite lengthy periods of observation,[77] but spontaneous cycling or other physiologic mucosal vascular change might give an impression of a contralateral response.

Initially decongestion is rapid and intense. It approaches completion in 15 minutes or less following adequate topical dosage of several different α-agonists, and combined resistance is almost halved in many healthy noses. It is reduced in much greater proportion in the majority of congested noses. Rapidity of response is similar, but duration of effect varies between decongestants from <1 to 8 hours,[83] and there seems little difference in response between healthy and coryzal noses.[84] In healthy noses response to decongestant is terminated by unilateral congestion that heralds return of the nasal cycle. Decongestion by vigorous exercise is even more rapid than by topical decongestant, and it is equally profound.[62]

As noted above, the contribution of inflammatory accumulations of extravascular fluid to nasal mucosal swelling and to airflow resistance is overshadowed in most cases by the vascular response to decongestant, and it appears that edema is not a major contributor to obstruction in the bulk of cases of inflammatory nasal disease.

Rhinitis Medicamentosa

There is often a disparity between therapeutic indications and actual use of topical nasal decongestants,[16] and the clinical impression that chronic use runs a risk of rhinitis medicamentosa is widely held. Yet a study of 6 weeks' treatment of healthy noses with xylometazoline did not reveal tachyphylaxis or any recognizable ciliary, eipthelial, or mucosal change.[146] Moreover, the sensation of rebound congestion that was experienced by the subjects was not confirmed by objective measurement.

The etiology of rhinitis medicamentosa that may result from chronic use of decongestant preparations is uncertain, but in addition to any part played by the decongestant, the preservative may be of importance. Rhinitis medicamentosa that is not resolved when decongestant treatment is discontinued could be due to its refractory nature, edema,[2] or persistence of the initiating obstructive condition. In such cases steroid therapy is usually helpful.

Decongestion can be achieved by weaker concentrations of decongestant than is customary in over-the-counter therapeutic preparations,[12] and there is merit in the Scandinavian practice of dispensing nasal decongestants as prescription medications in small, sterile quantities without preservative.

> **Clinical comment:** Rapid shrinking of inflamed mucosa by an α-agonist is predominantly the response of capacitance vessels and is uncharacteristic of edema or hypertrophy.

SUMMARY

A narrowed segment of the anterior nose forms the major resistor of the entire respiratory airway. It is a dynamic resistor with a length of several millimeters, shaped and stabilized by the bony piriform margin, compliant alar cartilages, and facial muscles. Erectile tissues of the lateral nasal wall and septum regulate nasal lumen and resistance to airflow, principally in the anterior nose. Erectile tissues are composed of tortuous masses of capacitance vessels that constrict in response to exercise, hypoxia, hypercarbia, and α-agonists and dilate in response to hyperventilation, cold air, irritants, and vasodilators. In addition, spontaneous reciprocal cycling of congestion and decongestion of erectile tissues takes place between sides. The cycle is overridden by lateral recumbent postures and by pressures applied to lateral body surfaces even in upright subjects. Lateral posture and pressure induce contralateral constriction and ipsilateral dilation.

Nasal obstruction is regularly troublesome in $>20\%$ of the population. It is a predominant inflammatory response of capacitance vessels to irritants, infective agents, and allergens. Similar vascular nasal obstruction of uncertain etiology is common also. Inflammatory congestion is reduced promptly by α-agonist medication and by topical steroid. Nasal congestion is associated with biochemical mediators, antidromic reflexes, and vasoactive neuropeptides. No humans escape nasal mucosal diseases, and many suffer significant consequences from them. When prevention or medical treatment is unsuccessful in reducing chronic obstructive nasal mucosal swelling, judicious surgical reduction of erectile tissue with specific attention to the valve region can relieve the cardinal symptom of obstruction without atrophic repercussions.

REFERENCES

1. Adamson P, Smith O, Cole P: The effect of cosmetic rhinoplasty on nasal patency. *Laryngoscope* 1990; 100(4):357–359.
2. Akerlund A, Bende M: Sustained use of xylometazoline nose drops aggravates vasomotor rhinitis. *Am J Rhinol* 1991; 5(4):157–160.
3. Almeida de CLR: Study of the adenovascular body of the posterior part of the nasal septum. *Arch Otolaryng* 1975; 101:344–347.
4. Andersson K-E, Bende M: Adrenoceptors in the control of human nasal mucosal blood flow. *Ann Otol Rhinol Laryngol* 1984; 93:179–182.
5. Angaard A: Capillary and shunt blood flow in the nasal mucosa of the cat. *Acta Otolaryngol (Stockh)* 1974; 78:418–422.
6. Arbour P, Bilgen E, Girardin M: La chirurgie de la valve liminaire etroite par la descente extranasale: Technique et explication biomechanique. *J Otolaryngol* 1976; 5(3):256–262.
7. Arbour P, Kern EB: Paradoxical nasal obstruction. *Can J Otolaryngol* 1975; 4(2):333–338.
8. Asakura K, Hoki K, Kataura A, et al: Respiration related movements of the nose in dogs. *Acta Otolaryngol (Stock)* 1986; 101:122–128.
9. Bachmann W, Legler U: Studies on the structure and function of the anterior section of the nose by means of luminal impressions. *Acta Otolaryngol (Stockh)* 1972; 73:433–442.
10. Batson OV: The venous networks of the nasal mucosa. *Ann Otol Rhinol Laryngol* 1954; 63(3):571–580.
11. Beickert P: Halbseitenrhythmus der vegetativen Innervation. *Arch Ohren Nasen Keilkopfheilkd* 1951; 157:404–407.
12. Bende M, Andersson K-E, Johansson C-J, et al: Dose-response relationship of a topical nasal decongestant: Phenylpropanolamine. *Acta Otolaryngol (Stock)* 1984; 98:543–547.
13. Bende M: Blood flow in human nasal mucosa (thesis). University Hospital, Lund, Sweden, 1983.
14. Bende M: The physiologic importance of the nasal mucosal vascular bed: A review. *Am J Rhinol* 1990; 5:189–191.
15. Berry RB: Nasal resistance before and after rhinoplasty. *Br J Plast Surg* 1981; 34:105–111.
16. Black MJ, Remsen KA: Rhinitis medicamentosa. *Can Med Assoc J* 1980; 122:881–884.
17. Bojsen-Moller F, Fahrenkrug J: Nasal swell-bodies and cyclic changes in the air passages of the rat and rabbit nose. *J Anat* 1971; 110(1):25–37.
18. Bohle MV, Karambelkar PV: Significance of nostrils in breathing. 1968; *Yoga Mimamsa* 10:1.
19. Briant TDR: Surgery of the nasal tip. *Can J Otolaryngol* 1973; 2(3):217–223.
20. Briant TDR: Management of severe septal deformities. *J Otolaryngol* 1985; 14(2):120–124.
21. Bridger GP, Proctor DF: Maximum nasal inspiratory flow and nasal resistance. *Ann Otol Rhinol Laryngol* 1970; 79(3):481–489.

22. Bridger GP: Physiology of the nasal valve. *Arch Otolaryngol* 1970; 92:543–553.
23. Broder I, Corey P, Cole P, et al: Comparison of health of occupants and characteristics of houses among control homes and homes insulated with urea formaldehyde foam. II. Initial health and house variables and exposure-response relationships. *Environ Res* 1988; 45:156–178.
24. Broder I, Higgins MW, Mathews KP, et al: Epidemiology of asthma and allergic rhinitis in a total community, Tecumseh, Michigan. *J Allergy Clin Immunol* 1974; 54:100–110.
25. Brown EA: Measurement of resistance of the nasal passages 1–3. *Rev Allerg* 1967; 21:472–857.
26. Cauna N: Blood and nerve supply of the nasal lining, in Proctor DF, Andersen IB (eds): *The Nose: Upper Airway Physiology and the Atmospheric Environment.* Amsterdam, Elsevier Biomedical Press, 1982.
27. Cawenberge van PB: Nasal cycle in children. *Arch Otolaryngol* 1984; 110:108–110.
28. Chaban R, Cole P, Naito K: Simulated septal deviations (2). *Arch Otolaryngol Head Neck Surg* 1988; 114:413–415.
29. Charlesworth EN, Iliopoulos O, MacDonald SM, et al: Cells and secretogogues involved in the human late-phase response. *Int Arch Allergy Appl Immunol* 1989; 88:50–53.
30. Cohen BM: The inter-relationship of respiratory functions of the nasal and lower airways. *Bull Physio-pathol Resp* 1971; 7:895–911.
31. Cole P: Stability of nasal airflow resistance. *Clin Otolaryngol* 1989; 14:177–182.
32. Cole P: Nasal turbinate function. *Can J Otolaryngol* 1973; 2(3):259–262.
33. Cole P: Modification of inspired air, in Mathew O, Sant'Ambrogio G (eds): *Respiratory Function of the Upper Airway.* New York, Marcel Dekker, 1988.
34. Cole P, Chaban R, Naito K, et al: The obstructive nasal septum: Effect of simulated deviations on nasal airflow resistance. *Arch Otolaryngol Head Neck Surg* 1988; 114:410–412.
35. Cole P, Haight JSJ, Cooper PW, et al: A computed tomographic study of nasal mucosa: effects of vasoactive substances. *J Otolaryngol* 1983; 12(1):58–60.
36. Cole P, Haight JSJ: Posture and the nasal cycle. *Ann Otol Rhinol Laryngol* 1986; 95:233–237.
37. Cole P, Haight JSJ: Posture and the nasal patency. *Am Rev Respir Dis* 1984; 129:351–354.
38. Cole P, Haight JSJ, Love L, et al: Dynamic components of nasal resistance. *Am Rev Respir Dis* 1985; 132:1229–1232.
39. Cole P, Haight JSJ, Naito K, et al: Magnetic resonance imaging of the nasal airways. *Am J Rhinol* 1989; 3(2):63–67.
40. Cole P: Upper respiratory airflow, in Proctor DF, Andersen IB (eds): *The Nose: Upper Airway Physiology and the Atmospheric Environment.* Amsterdam, Elsevier Biomedical Press, 1982.

41. Cole P, Forsyth R, Haight JSJ: Effects of cold air and exercise on nasal patency. *Ann Otol Rhinol Laryngol* 1983; 92(2):196–198.
42. Connell JT: Nasal disease, in Settipane GA (ed): *Rhinitis.* Providence, RI, OceanSide Publications, 1991.
43. Cornelissen G, Halberg F, Tarquini B: Ultradian rhythms: A neglected yet promising domain of the rhythm spectrum, in Fanfani M, Tarquini B (eds): *Reference Values and Chronobiology* (XV World Congress of Anatomic and Clinical Pathology, Florence 1989).
44. Cottle MH: The structure and function of the nasal vestibule. *Arch Otolaryngol* 1955; 62:173–181.
45. Courtiss EH, Goldwyn RL: Resection of obstructing inferior nasal turbinates. *Plast Reconstr Surg* 1978; 62(2):249–257.
46. Courtiss EH, Goldwyn RL: The effects of nasal surgery on airflow. *Plast and Reconstr Surg* 1983; 72(1):9–18.
47. Crysdale WS, Cole P, Emery P: Cephalometric radiographs, nasal airway resistance and adenoidectomy. *J Otolaryngol* 1985; 14(2):92–94.
48. Dallimore NS, Eccles R: Changes in human nasal resistance associated with exercise, hyperventilation and rebreathing. *Acta Otolaryngol (Stockh)* 1977; 84:416–421.
49. Davis DL, Hertzman AB: Analysis of vascular reactions in the nasal mucosa with the photoelectric plethysmograph. *Ann Otol Rhinol Laryngol* 1957; 66(2):622–640.
50. Dawes PJD: The early complications of inferior turbinectomy. *J Laryngol Otol* 1987; 101:1136–1139.
51. DesPrez JD, Kiehn CL: Valvular obstruction of the nasal airway. *Plast Reconstr Surg* 1975; 56(3):307–313.
52. Dishock van HAE: Inspiratory nasal resistance. *Acta Otolaryngol (Stockh)* 1942; 30:431–439.
53. Dishoek van HAE: Electogramm der Nasenflogelmuskeln. *Acta Otolaryngol (Stockh)* 1937; 25:293–295.
54. Drake AF, Keall H, Vig PS, et al: Clinical nasal obstruction and objective respiratory mode determination. *Ann Otol Rhinol Laryngol* 1988; 97:397–402.
55. Drettner B: Vascular reactions of the human nasal mucosa on exposure to cold. *Acta Otolaryngol (Stockh)* 1961; 166(suppl):1–109.
56. Eccles R: Studies on the nasal cycle in the immobilized pig. *J Physiol* 1975; 247:1P.
57. Eccles R, Lee RL: Nasal vasomotor oscillations in the cat associated with the respiratory rhythm. *Acta Otolaryngol (Stockh)* 1981; 92:357–361.
58. Eccles R: Rhinomanometry and nasal challenge, in Mackay IS, Bull TR (eds): *Otolaryngology-Rhinology,* ed 5. London, Butterworth, 1987.
59. Ferres HM: Effect of pressure on sweating. *J Physiol* 1958; 143:39.
60. Finger TE, Getchell ML, Getchell TV, et al: in Attector and effector Functions of peptidergic innervation of the nasal cavity, Green, Mason R, Kare MR (eds): *Chemical Senses. Irritation,* vol 2. New York, Marcel Dekker, 1990, pp 1-20.

61. Fior R, Veljak C: Septum dislocation in the newborn: A long-term follow-up. *Rhinology* 1990; 28(3):159–162.
62. Forsyth RD, Cole P, Shephard RJ: Exercise and nasal patency. *J Appl Physiol* 1983; 55(3):860–865.
63. Francis D: *Straight.* England, Penguin Books Ltd., 1989, 253–257.
64. Franklin W: Controlled studies of immunotherapy in allergic rhinitis: A critical review, in Settipane GA (ed): *Rhinitis.* Providence, RI, OceanSide Publications Inc, 1991.
65. Gilbert AN, Rosenwasser AM: Biological rhythmicity of nasal airway patency: A re-examination of the nasal cycle. *Acta Otolaryngol (Stockh)* 1987; 104:180–186.
66. Golding-Wood PH: Vidian neurectomy: its results and complications. *Laryngoscope* 1973; 83(10):1673–1683.
67. Goode RL: Surgery of the incompetent nasal valve. *Laryngoscope* 1985; 95:546–555.
68. Gray LP: Deviated nasal septum incidence and etiology. *Ann Otol Rhinol Laryngol* 1978; 87(3)(Suppl 50):1–20.
69. Gray LP: Results of 310 cases of rapid maxillary expansion selected for medical reasons. *J Laryngol Otol* 1975; 89:601–614.
70. Grymer LF, Hilberg O, Pedersen OF, et al: Acoustic rhinometry: Values from adults with subjective normal nasal patency. *Rhinology* 1991; 29(1):35–47.
71. Gwaltney JM, Hayden FG: The nose and infection, in Proctor DF, Andersen IB (eds): *The Nose: Upper Airway Physiology and the Atmospheric Environment.* Amsterdam, Elsevier Biomedical Press, 1982.
72. Haight JSJ, Cole P: Is the nasal cycle an artefact? The role of asymmetrical postures. *Laryngoscope* 1989; 99(5):538–541.
73. Haight JSJ, Cole P: Nasal resistance after lateral recumbency. *J Otolaryngol* 1986; 15(Suppl 16):9–13.
74. Haight JSJ, Cole P, Cooper PW, et al: The choana and nasal obstruction. *J Otolaryngol* 1985; 14(2):99–102.
75. Haight JSJ, Cole P: Reciprocating nasal airflow resistances. *Acta Otolaryngol (Stockh)* 1984; 97:93–98.
76. Haight JSJ, Cole P: The site and function of the nasal valve. *Laryngoscope* 1983; 93(1):49–55.
77. Haight JSJ, Cole P: Nasal responses to local unilateral stimuli in man. *Rhinology* 1983; 21:67–72.
78. Haight JSJ, Gardiner GW: Nasal cryo-surgery and cautery: Should the septum be treated and is a diagnosis relevant? *J Otolaryngol* 1989; 18:144–150.
79. Haight JSJ, Cole P: Topographical anatomy of the pressure points that alter nasal resistance. *J Otolaryngol* 1986; 15(Suppl 16):14–20.
80. Haight JSJ, Cole P: Blockade of the nasal response to asymmetrical body pressures. *J Otolaryngol* 1986; 15(Suppl 16).
81. Hairfield WM, Warren DW, Hinton VA, et al: Inspiratory and expiratory effects of nasal breathing. *Cleft Pal J* 1987; 24(3):183–189.

82. Hales JRS: Regulation of the cutaneous circulation. *Fed Proc* 1986; 45:2844–2846.
83. Hamilton LH: Effect of topical decongestants on nasal airway resistance. *Current Ther Res* 1978; 24(3):261–268.
84. Hamilton LH: Effect of xylometazoline nasal spray on nasal conductance in subjects with coryza. *J Otolaryngol* 1981; 10(2):109–116.
85. Hasegawa M: Nasal cycle and postural variations in nasal resistance. *Ann Otol Rhinol Laryngol* 1982; 91(1):112–114.
86. Hasegawa M, Saito Y: Postural variations in nasal resistance and symptomatology in allergic rhinitis. *Acta Otolaryngol (Stockh)* 1979; 88:268–272.
87. Havas TE, Cole P, Gullane PJ, et al: The nasal cycle after laryngectomy. *Acta Otolaryngol (Stockh)* 1987; 103:111–116.
88. Heetderks DL: Observations on the reaction of the normal nasal mucous membrane. *Am J Med Sci* 1927; 174:231–244.
89. Heyden R: The respiratory function in laryngectomized patients. *Acta Otolaryngol Suppl (Stockh)* 1950; 85:1–60.
90. Hildebrandt G: Untersuchungen uber den Zeitigkeit Rhythmus der Nasen Atmung (thesis). Phillips Universitat z. Marburg, 1970.
91. Holmes TH, Goodell H, Wolf S, et al: *The Nose: An Experimental Study of Reaction Within the Nose in Human Subjects During Various Life Experiences.* Springfield, Ill, CC Thomas, 1950.
92. Hudgel DW, Robertson DW: Nasal resistance during wakefulness and sleep in normal man. *Acta Otolaryngol (Stockh)* 1984; 98:130–135.
93. Jones AS, Wight RG, Kabil Y, et al: Predicting the outcome of submucosal diathermy to the inferior turbinates. *Clin Otolaryngol* 1989; 14:41–44.
94. Jones AS, Wight RG, Stevens JC, et al: The nasal valve: A physiological and clinical study. *J Laryngol Otol* 1988; 102:1089–1094.
95. Jones AS, Lancer JM, Moir, AA, et al: The effect of submucosal diathermy to the inferior turbinates on nasal resistance to airflow in allergic and vasomotor rhinitis. *Clin Otolaryngol* 1985; 10:249–252.
96. Jones AS, Lancer JM: Does submucosal diathermy to the inferior turbinates reduce nasal resistance to airflow in the long term? *J Laryngol Otol* 1987; 101:448–451.
97. Jonson B, Rundcrantz H: Posture and pressure within the internal juglar vein. *Acta Otolaryngol (Stockh)* 1969; 68:271–275.
98. Juto JE, Lundberg C: Variation in nasal congestion during rest. *Acta Otolaryngol (Stockh)* 1984; 98:136–139.
99. Kaliner M: in *Management of Allergy in the 1990's.* Toronto, Hans Huber Publishers, 1989.
100. Kasperbauer JL, Kern EB: Nasal valve physiology implications in nasal surgery. *Otolaryngol Clin N Am* 1987; 20(4):699–719.
101. Kawase T: Further studies on pressure sweat reflexes. *Jap J Physiol* 1950; 3:1–9.
102. Kayser R: Die exacte Messung der Luftdurchgangikeit der Nase. *Arch Laryngol* 1895; 3:101–120.

103. Kellerhals B, Schlageter J: Cryosurgery in vasomotor rhinopathy: experimental histopathology. *ORL J Otorhinolaryngol Relat Spec* 1976; 38:157–163.
104. Keuning J: On the nasal cycle. Thesis, 1968; University of Leiden, Netherlands.
105. Klein R, Pilon O, Prosser S, et al: Nasal airflow asymmetries and human performance. *Biol Psychol* 1986; 23:127–137.
106. Knowles MR, et al: Nasal secretions: role of epithelial ion transport, in Mygind N, Pipkorn U (eds): *Allergic and Vasomotor Rhinitis: Pathophysiological Aspects.* Copenhagen, Munksgaard, 1987.
107. Kosoy J: Nasal surgery and airway patency. *Laryngoscope* 1979; 89(10):1655–1680.
108. Kuno Y: *Human Perspiration.* Springfield, Ill, CC Thomas, 1956.
109. Lacourt G, Polgar G: Interaction between nasal and pulmonary resistance in newborn infants. *J Appl Physiol* 1971; 30(6):870–873.
110. Lancer JM, Jones AS: The Francis alae nasi prop and nasal resistance to airflow. *J Laryngol* 1986; 100:539–541.
111. Leclerc J, Doyle WJ, Karnavas WJ: The relationship between the nasal cycle and axillary sweat production. *Rhinology* 1987; 24(4):249–257.
112. Leiberman A, Cole P, Corey M, et al: Otolaryngological and rhinomanometric findings in cystic fibrosis. *Am J Rhinol* 1991; 5(2):61–65.
113. Lenders H, Persig W: Diagnostic value of acoustic rhinometry: patients with allergic and vasomotor rhinitis compared with normal controls. *Rhinology* 1990; 28:5–16.
114. Lillie HI: Some practical considerations of the physiology of the upper respiratory tract. *J Iowa Med Soc* 1923; 13:403–408.
115. Lung M, Wang JCC: Nasal blood flow and airway resistance. *Ann Otol Rhinol Laryngol* 1985; 94(2):198–201.
116. Lung M, Wang JCC: Arterial supply, venous drainage and collateral circulation in the nose of the anaesthetized dog. *J Physiol* 1987; 391:57–70.
117. Lunteren van E, Haxhiu MA, Cherniak S: Respiratory changes in nasal muscle length. *J Appl Physiol* 1985; 59(2):453–458.
118. Lunteren van E, Strohl KP: Striated respiratory muscles of the upper airway, in Mathew OP, Sant'Ambrogio G (eds): *Respiratory Function of the Upper Airway.* New York, Marcel Dekker, 1988.
119. Mabry RL: Uses and misuses of corticosteroids and cromalin. *Am J Rhinol* 1991; 5(3):121–124.
120. Malling HJ: New ideas in allergen-specific immunotherapy. *Am J Rhinol* 1990; 4(4):155–158.
121. Malm L: Resistance and capacitance vessels in the nasal mucosa. *Rhinology* 1975; 13:85–89.
122. Martinez SA, Nissen AJ, Stock CR, et al: Nasal turbinate resection for relief of nasal obstruction. *Laryngoscope* 1983; 93:871–875.
123. McCaffrey TV, Kern EB: Response of the nasal airway to hypercapnia and hypoxia in man. *Ann Otol Rhinol Laryngol* 1979; 88:247–252.
124. Mertz JS, McCaffrey TV, Kern EB: Objective evaluation of anterior septal surgical reconstruction. *Otolaryngol Head Neck Surg* 1984; 92(3):308–311.

125. Mink PJ: Die Rolle des karvenosen Gewebes in der Nase. *Arch Laryngol* 1916; 30:47–65.
126. Moore GF, Freeman TJ, Ogren FP, et al: Extended follow-up of total inferioir turbinate resection for relief of chronic nasal obstruction. *Laryngoscope* 1985; 95:1095–1099.
127. Mygind N: Immunotherapy, in *Nasal Allergy.* Oxford, Blackwell Scientific Publications, 1978.
128. Mygind N: Morphology of the upper airway epithelium, in Proctor DF, Andersen IB (eds): *The nose: Upper airway physiology and the atmospheric environment.* Amsterdam, Elsevier Biomedical Press, 1982.
129. Mygind N, Lowenstein H: Allergy and other environmental factors, in Proctor DF, Anderson IB (eds): *The Nose: Upper Airway Physiology and the Atmospheric Environment.* Amsterdam, Elsevier Biomedical Press, 1982.
130. Mygind N, Sorensen H, Pedersen CB: The nasal mucosa during long-term treatment with beclomethasone diproprionate aerosol. *Acta Otolaryngol (Stockh)* 1978; 85:437–443.
131. Mygind N, Anggard A, Druce HM: Definition, classification and terminology, in Mygind N, Weeke B (eds): *Allergic and Vasomotor Rhinitis: Clinical Aspects.* Copenhagen, Munksgaard, 1985.
132. Naclerio RM, Okuda M, Pipkorn U: Late phase allergic reactions in the nose, in Mygind N, Weeke B (eds): *Allergic and Vasomotor Rhinitis: Clinical Aspects.* Copenhagen, Munksgaard, 1985.
133. Naito K, Iwata S, Kondo M, et al: The influence of the normal turbinate mucosa on nasal airflow. *Eur Arch Otorhinolaryngol* 1990; 247:174–175.
134. Negus VE: *The Comparative Anatomy and Physiology of the Nose and Paranasal Sinuses.* London, Livingstone, 1958.
135. Odetoyinbo O: Complications following total inferior turbinectomy: Fact or myth? *Clin Otolaryngol* 1987; 12:361–363.
136. Ogura JH, Stocksted P: Rhinomanometry in some rhinologic diseases. *Laryngoscope* 1958; 68:2001–2014.
137. Ogura JH, Harvey JE: Nasopulmonary mechanics: Experimental evidence of the influence of the upper airway on the lower. *Acta Otolaryngol (Stockh)* 1971; 71:123–132.
138. Ohki M, Hasegawa M, Kurita N, et al: Effects of exercise on nasal resistance and nasal blood flow. *Acta Otolaryngol (Stockh)* 1987; 108:328–333.
139. Ohki M, Hasegawa M, Sakuma A: Exercise induced nasal obstruction in patients with allergic rhinitis. *Am J Rhinol* 1989; 3(1):1–4.
140. Olsson P: Studies of blood flow in human nasal mucosa (thesis). University Hospital, Lund, Sweden, 1986.
141. Ophir D, Elad Y: Effects of steam inhalation on nasal patency and symptoms in patients with the common cold. *Am J Otolaryngol* 1987; 8(3):149–153.
142. Ophir D, Shapira A, Marshak G: Total inferior turbinectomy for nasal airway obstruction. *Arch Otolaryngol* 1985; 3:93–95.
143. Parker LP, Crysdale WS, Cole P, et al: Rhinomanometry in children. *Int J Ped Otorhinolaryngol* 1989; 17:127–137.

144. Paulsson B, Bende M, Ohlin P: Nasal mucosal blood flow at rest and during exercise. *Acta Otolaryngol (Stockh)* 1985; 99:140–143.
145. Petruson B: Snoring can be reduced when the nasal airflow is increased by the nasal dilator Nazovent. *Arch Otolaryngol Head Neck Surg* 1981; 116:462–464.
146. Petruson B: Function and structure of the nasal mucosa after 6 weeks' use of nose drops. *Acta Otolaryngol (Stockh)* 1982; 94:563–569.
147. Phillips JJ: The cosmetic effects of submucous resection. *Clin Otolaryngol* 1991; 16:179–181.
148. Pollock RA, Rohrich RJ: Inferior turbinate surgery: An adjunct to successful treatment of nasal obstruction in 408 patients. *Plast Reconstr Surg* 1984; 74(2):227–234.
149. Principato JJ, Ozenberger JM: Cyclical changes in nasal resistance. *Arch Otolaryngol* 1970; 91:71–77.
150. Proctor DF: Nasal physiology in intranasal drug administration, in Chen YW (ed): *Transnasal Systemic Medication.* Amsterdam, Elsevier, 1985, pp 101–106.
151. Ralston HJ, Kerr WJ: Vascular responses of nasal mucosa to thermal stimuli: With some observations on skin temperature. *Am J Physiol* 1945; 144:305–310.
152. Richerson HB, Seebohm PM: Nasal airway response to exercise. *J Allergy* 1968; 41:269–284.
153. Rothe CF: Reflex control of veins and vascular capacitance. *Physiol Rev* 1983; 63(4):1281–1342.
154. Rundcrantz H: Posture and congestion of nasal mucosa in allergic rhinitis. *Acta Otolaryngol (Stockh)* 1964; 58:283–287.
155. Rundcrantz H: Postural variations of nasal patency. *Acta Otolaryngol (Stockh)* 1969; 68:435–443.
156. Santiago-Diez de Bonilla J, McCaffrey TV, Kern EB: The nasal valve: A rhinomanometric evaluation of maximum nasal inspiratory flow and pressure curves. *Ann Otol Rhinol Laryngol* 1986; 95:229–232.
157. Sasaki CT, Suzuki M, Fukuda H, et al: Dilator naris muscle. *Ann Otol Rhinol Laryngol* 1977; 86(1):362–370.
158. Sasaki CT, Mann DG: Dilator naris function. *Arch Otolaryngol* 1976; 102:365–367.
159. Schuman K, Laniado K: Der Einfluss einer Septumdeviation auf die Lungenfunktion. *HNO* 1981; 26:6–9.
160. Siegel SC: Topical corticosteroids in the management of rhinitis, in Settipane GA (ed): *Rhinitis.* Providence, RI, OceanSide Publications, 1991.
161. Settipane GA: New England and regional allergy proceedings, in Settipane GA (ed): *Rhinitis.* Providence, RI, OceanSide Publications, 1991.
162. Shannahoff-Khalsa D: Lateralized rhythms of the central and autonomic nervous systems. *Intern J Psychophysiol* 1991, in press.
163. Shannahoff-Khalsa D: Stress technology medicine: A new paradigm for

stress and considerations for self regulation, in Brown M, Koob G, Rivier C (eds): *Stress: Neurobiology and Neuroendocrinology.* New York, Marcel Dekker, 1991.

164. Singh B, Chhina GA: Some reflections on ancient Indian physiology, in Keswani NH, Manchandra SK (eds): *The Science of Medicine and Physiological Concepts in Ancient and Mediaeval India.* New Delhi, 26th International Congress of Physiological Sciences, 1974.
165. Slavit DH, Lipton RJ, Kern EB: Rhinolift operation in the treatment of the aging nose. *Otolaryngol Head Neck Surg* 1990; 103:462–467.
166. Smith O, Adamson PA, Tropper G, et al: The role of partial turbinectomy in septorhinoplasty: A prospective randomized trial. *Proc 5th Int Symp Fac Plast Reconstr Surg* 1990.
167. Stocksted P, Gutierrez C: The nasal passage following rhinoplastic surgery. *J Laryngol Otol* 1983; 97:49–54.
168. Stocksted P: The physiologic cycle of the nose under normal and pathologic conditions. *Acta Otolaryngol (Stockh)* 1952; 42:175–179.
169. Stocksted P: Rhinometric measurements for determination of the nasal cycle. *Acta Otolaryngol (Suppl) (Stockh)* 1953; 109:159–175.
170. Strohl KP: Upper airway muscles of respiration. *Am Rev Respir Dis* 1981; 124:211–213.
171. Sulsenti G, Palma P: The nasal valve area: structure, function, clinics and treatment. *Acta Otolaryngol Ital* 1989; suppl 22:3–25.
172. Sulsenti G, Palma P: A new technique for functional surgery of the nasal valve area. *Rhinology* 1989; suppl 10:1–19.
173. Swift DL, Proctor DF: Access of air to the respiratory tract, in Proctor DF, Reid LM (eds): *Respiratory Defense Mechanisms.* New York, Marcel Dekker, 1977.
174. Tagaki K, Kobayasi S: Skin pressure-vegetative reflex. *Acta Medica et Biol* 1955; 4:3–57.
175. Tagaki K, Sakuri T: A sweat reflex due to pressure on the body surface. *Jap J Physiol* 1950; 1:22–28.
176. Tatum AL: The effect of deficient and excessive pulmonary ventilation on nasal volume. *Am J Physiol* 1923; 64–65:229–233.
177. Timms DJ: The reduction of nasal airway resistance by rapid maxillary expansion and its effect on respiratory disease. *J Laryngol Otol* 1984; 98:357–362.
178. Tolley NS, Parker A, Hawthorne M, et al: Critical investigation of the method of inferior turbinectomy. *Clin Otolaryngol* 1989; 14:268.
179. Tschalussov MA: *Arch ges Physiol.* 1913; 51:523–542. Quoted by Tatum, 1923.
180. Vanio-Mattila J: Correlation of nasal symptoms and signs in random sampling study. *Acta Otolaryngol (Suppl) (Stockh)* 1974; 318:1–48.
181. Vishnudevananda S: *The Complete Illustrated Book of Yoga.* New York, Bell Publishing, 1959.
182. Walker DA, Turvey TA, Warren DW: Alteration in nasal respiration and

nasal airway size following superior repositioning of the maxilla. *J Oral Maxillofac Surg* 1988; 46:276–281.
183. Warren DW, Hershy GH, Turvey TA, et al: The nasal airway following maxillary expansion. *Am J Orthod Dentofacial Orthop* 1987; 91:111–116.
184. Weeke ER, Pedersen PA, Backman A, et al: Epidemiology, in Mygind N, Weeke B (eds): *Allergic and Vasomotor Rhinitis: Clinical Aspects.* Copenhagen, Munksgaard, 1985.
185. Weinkauf FJ, Rowland GC: Patient conditions at the primary-care level; A commentary on resource allocation. *Ontario Med Rev* 1992; 59(1):11–15.
186. Wengraf CL, Gleeson MJ, Siodlak MZ: The stuffy nose: A comparative study of two common methods of treatment. *Clin Otolaryngol* 1986; 11:61–68.
187. Werntz DA, Bickford RJ, Shannahoff-Khalsa DS: Selective hemispheric stimulation by unilateral forced nostril breathing. *Hum Neurobiol* 1987; 6:165–171.
188. Werntz DA, Bickford RJ, Bloom FE, Shannahoff-Khalsa DS: Alternating cerebral hemispheric activity and lateralization of autonomic nervous function. *Hum Neurobiol* 1983; 2:39–43.
189. White BC, Woodside DG, Cole P: Effect of rapid maxillary expansion on nasal airway resistance. *J Otolaryngol* 1989; 18(4):137–143.
190. Widdicombe JG: The physiology of the nose. *Clin Chest Med* 1986; 7(2):159–170.
191. Widdicombe JG: Nasal and pharyngeal reflexes, in Mathew OP, Sant'Ambrogio G (eds): *Respiratory Function of the Upper Airway.* New York, Marcel Dekker, 1988.
192. Widdicombe JG, Sant'Ambrogio G, Mathew OP: Nerve receptors of the upper airway, in Mathew OP, Sant'Ambrogio G (eds): *Respiratory Function of the Upper Airway.* New York, Marcel Dekker, 1988.
193. Widdicombe JG, Wells UM: Airway secretions, in Proctor DF, Andersen IB (eds): *The Nose: Upper Airway Physiology and the Atmospheric Environment.* Amsterdam, Elsevier Biomedical Press, 1982.
194. Widdicombe JG: The regulation of bronchial calibre, in Caro CG (ed): *Advances in Respiratory Physiology.* Baltimore, Williams & Wilkins, 1966, 48–82.
195. Wight RG, Jones AS, Beckingham E: Trimming of the inferior turbinates: A prospective long-term study. *Clin Otolaryngol* 1990; 15:347–350.
196. Wustrow F: Schwellkorper am Septum nasi. *Z Anat Entwicklunggesch* 1951; 116:139–142.
197. Wyllie JW, Kern EB, O'Brien PC, Hyatt RE: Alterations in pulmonary function associated with artificial nasal obstruction. *Otolarngology* 1976; 27:535–537.
198. Zinreich SJ, Kennedy DW, Kumar AJ, et al: MR imaging of normal nasal cycle: Comparison with sinus pathology. *J Comput Assist Tomogr* 1988; 12(6):1014–1019.
199. Zohar Y, Talmi YP, Strauss M, et al: Ozena revisited. *J Otolaryngol* 1990; 19(5):345–349.

SUGGESTED READING

1. Mathew OP, Sant' Ambrogio G (eds): *Respiratory Function of the Upper Airways.* New York, Marcel Dekker, 1988.
2. Mygind N, Pipkorn U (eds): *Allergic and Vasomotor Rhinitis: Pathophysiological Aspects.* Copenhagen, Munksgaard, 1987.
3. Mygind N, Weeke B (eds): *Allergic and Vasomotor Rhinitis: Clinical Aspects.* Copenhagen, Munksgaard, 1985.
4. Proctor DF, Anderson I (eds): *The Nose: Upper Airway Physiology and the Atmospheric Environment.* Amsterdam, Elsevier Biomedical Press, 1982.
5. Settipane GA (ed): *Rhinitis.* Providence, RI, OceanSide Publications, 1991.

CHAPTER 2

The Mouth and Throat

THE MOUTH AS A RESPIRATORY ORGAN

In addition to its functions of mastication, swallowing, and articulation, the mouth provides a parallel airway with the nose and, as a respiratory passage, it can bypass the nasal airways partially or completely. Indeed, without the alternative of an oral airway, patients with rhinitis might be in as serious danger of asphyxiation as patients with epiglottitis.

Oral structures are necessarily mobile, but in awake subjects, compliance of these structures with inspiratory airflow pressures or with gravity has little effect on oral airway patency. That is regulated by voluntary muscle positioning of the mandible, tongue, soft palate, and lips. In sleep compliant obstruction of the oral airway can occur and dependence on nasal patency is increased, as described later in this chapter.

Buccal, lingual, gingival, and palatal mucosa and dental surfaces exposed to the respiratory airstream during periods of oral breathing provide warm, moist areas available for air conditioning (see Chapter 3). These surfaces, moistened by secretions of major and minor salivary glands, comprise a substantial area that approaches the dimensions of the nasal-airway mucosa. Distribution of saliva is aided by mobility of the oral structures. In contrast with the nasal mucosa, the lack of a mucociliary system makes frequent mechanical distribution of moisture necessary to prevent parching of the mouth by the inspiratory airstream during lengthy periods of oral breathing.

The labial aperture provides an oral airflow regulator. It is a resistor, and its variable cross section is the major determinant of transoral airflow resistance; lip separation of only a few millimeters can reduce respiratory airway pressures markedly.[28] As with the nasal valve, the resistor is situated at an airway portal. The essential respiratory function of physiologic resistors at both oral and nasal airway portals is discussed in Chapter 3.

MOUTH BREATHING

The Oral Airway

In healthy adults the mouth provides an airway for about half the respiratory airflow during speech,[5] singing, and vigorous exercise.[68, 70] In addition, in healthy subjects at rest, oral breathing occurs spontaneously with irregular frequency and duration, often during periods of concentration, preoccupation, or emotional disturbance. Both an open-mouth posture and oronasal breathing are too commonplace to be regarded as necessarily abnormal; but continued mouth breathing for protracted periods, from habit, obstruction, or other causes, is a source of discomfort unless the mucosa is repeatedly moistened – and it may lead to pathologic consequences. Habitual mouth breathing can become very firmly established, and in many cases it is not rectified by relief of chronic nasal obstruction.[92]

It is widely taught that nasal breathing is obligatory in neonates, but observations indicate that these infants can resort readily to sustained and effective mouth breathing both spontaneously and in response to acute artificial nasal obstruction.[67, 85, 98] However, severe nasal obstruction may cause difficulties in suckling. Furthermore, cyanotic incidents reported in an infant with traumatic chronic nasal obstruction imply that the oral airway may not have provided complete compensation.[66] Infants whose history suggests "near-miss sudden death syndrome" behave no differently from other infants in response to acute nasal occlusion.[84] In cases of severe nasal obstruction in patients of all ages, adequate oral-airway function is a lifeline, and it may become tenuous in sleep (discussed later).

Oronasal Breathing

If the burden of nasal breathing becomes intolerable, it is shared with the parallel oral airway; but measurements have shown that this airway, too, is resistive to respiratory airflow. When lips and mandible are spontaneously positioned, oral resistance to respiratory airflow assumes a similar magnitude to that of the healthy nose. Furthermore, transoral resistance to respiratory airflow is reduced by 80% to 90% on widening of the spontaneous aperture of the lips and teeth by only a few millimeters (Fig 2–1).[9, 28] It appears, therefore, that the contribution of the palatoglossal segment of the airway to transoral respiratory airflow resistance is small, and as with transnasal resistance, the major portion of transoral resistance is localized to the vestibular region.[9]

Video studies have demonstrated mouths of participants entering the final kilometers of a 10 km run[69] to be only partially open, not maximally patent, enabling an oral resistor to play a role in regulating oronasal distribution of respiratory airflow and in conditioning inspiratory air (see Chapter 3, "Air Conditioning"). Measurements obtained from exercising subjects have shown that a majority of healthy young adults switch from nasal to oronasal breathing as resting ventilation is quadrupled (to about 35 L/min).

The nasal fraction of respiratory airflow decreases to 60% at the switch point, and it decreases further to 40% as ventilation approaches 100 L/min.[8, 68, 70] In other words, although the mucovascular component of nasal

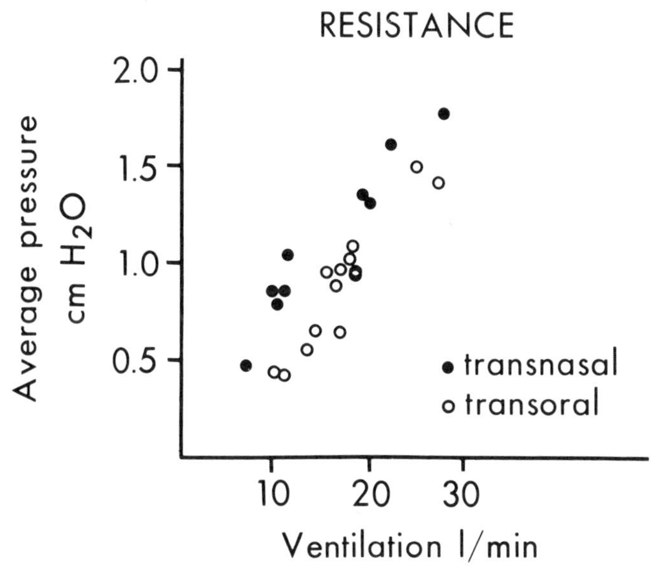

FIG 2–1.

Transoral and transnasal pressures in subjects breathing at different ventilations exclusively through either the nose or the spontaneously positioned mouth. Note similarity of resistances. (From Cole P, Forsyth R, Haight JSJ: Respiratory resistance of the oral airway. *Am Rev Respir Dis* 1982; 125:363. Used by permission.)

resistance is diminished by exercise (Chapter 1 and Fig 1–19), increasing exercise brings about even greater diminution of oral resistance, resulting in augmentation of the oral fraction of oronasal breathing from 40% to 60%.

An additional series of acute experiments has shown that a majority of healthy young adults switch to oronasal breathing as artificial resistances are added sequentially to the nasal airway and total nasal resistances approach 0.5 Pa/cm^3/sec (Forte and Cole, unpublished, 1988). In these experiments, each group included about 10% chronic "mouth breathers" at rest and a similar proportion of subjects who persisted in exclusive nasal breathing under conditions of quite severe exercise[68, 70] or nasal obstruction.

Consequences of Oronasal Breathing

In sleep and other forms of diminished consciousness (see below), the respiratory roles of the nose and mouth are changed, with dependence on nasal patency being increased. Yet nasal obstruction of either abnormal mucosal or structural origin is exacerbated by recumbency.

The oral airway combines characteristics of nose and pharynx. Oral resistance is localized to the spontaneously positioned oral vestibule in awake subjects. It is of similar magnitude to resistance in the valve region of the nasal vestibule. It is increased in sleep and even when the labial aperture is patent and the mouth provides an airway, it is a precarious one. Relaxation of voluntary muscle tone and effects of gravity and airflow pressures on flaccid tissues of the tongue, palate, cheeks, and lips can result in marked elevation of oral-airway resistance.[74, 75] Oral breathing in sleep is frequently accompanied by snoring or other obstructive sounds, and it leads also to complaints of dry mouth and pharyngeal discomfort.

Nasal packing following surgery or for control of epistaxis is not without respiratory complications that are exacerbated by sleep and by sedatives, especially in older patients. Several investigators have recorded sleep apneas and disordered blood gases in such cases.[100]

The consequences of an impaired nasal airway are compensated by oronasal breathing in the awake subject, but, as described above, oral compensation is less assured in sleep. Disordered breathing, hypopneas, apneas, and fragmented sleep patterns are found in severely nasally obstructed subjects who are otherwise healthy.[74, 97] The pathologic implications of nasal obstruction in sleeping patients deserve wider recognition than they are generally afforded.

Chronic Mouth Breathing

Chronic mouth breathing is a common complaint in adult patients, but when adults complain about mouth breathing in children the term may be inaccurate. It is commonly applied to subjects whose lips remain chronically separated while they are in a resting state and does not necessarily describe the route or distribution of respiratory air. Moreover, nasal breathing is seldom replaced but it is frequently supplemented by oral breathing. Some 10% to 15% of adults[103] and a larger proportion of children are reported to be persistent "mouth breathers" at rest.[51]

In addition to creating a vacant expression and contributing to gingival disease, chronic mouth breathing is widely, but not universally, regarded as an important etiological factor in developmental abnormalities of dentition and facial structure in children. There is much clinical,[61, 114] experimental[25, 26] and statistical[113] evidence to support this view. Nevertheless, the relative importance of genetic and environmental influences on upper-airway dimensions, mode of breathing, and dentofacial development have not been established conclusively,[46, 73, 102, 104] and subjective criteria have led to differing views.[29]

The clinician, in many cases an otolaryngologist, is often called on to make recommendations and to undertake responsibility for therapy in cases of suspected upper-airway malfunction that may have been suggested by transient or chronic upper-airway obstruction, chronic "mouth breathing," or abnormalities of facial and dental development. There is little doubt that persistent upper-airway obstruction warrants treatment on its own merits, but the reluctance of orthodontists to undertake corrective therapy without assurance of the adequacy of upper-airway respiratory function presents medical practitioners with a common diagnostic dilemma. Persuasive evidence supports the view that there is an unfavorable relationship between upper-airway impairment and dentofacial morphology; and although it is reasonable to expect that, in many cases, spontaneous resolution of airway disability will take place over time (e.g., adenoid hypertrophy or inflammatory nasal obstruction), as fortunate a course of dentofacial maldevelopment cannot be anticipated with the same degree of optimism. These considerations usually influence the urgency of therapeutic decisions. Accurate assessment of nasal patency and oronasal airflow are necessary to provide a firm basis for rational therapy and an adjunct to quality control. The limitations of clinical assessment by history and inspection and the merits of quantitative evaluation of nasal airflow resistances and of oronasal breathing are discussed in Chapter 4.

Clinical comment: Withholding intervention for a lengthy period in expectation of spontaneous resolution of chronic upper-airway obstruction is seldom justified if obstructive malfunction is confirmed. Objective confirmation and follow-up contribute to diagnosis, quality control, and the accuracy of etiological data.

Upper-Airway Resistances and Oronasal Breathing

Exclusive nasal breathing in awake subjects at rest persists spontaneously over a wide range of nasal resistances in children and adults. By contrast, in many cases of reported "chronic mouth breathing," rhinomanometry reveals an unobstructed nasal airway. Moreover, fully one fourth of the pediatric patients referred to us as "mouth breathers" are actually 100% nose breathers despite the presence of a labial gap at the time of objective assessment (Chapter 4, "Objective Assessment of Oronasal Breathing"). Neither the open mouth nor mouth breathing is a reliable indicator of nasal resistance, and vice versa, but oral and nasal resistances each play a part in the regulation of respiratory airflow distribution between these parallel airways during oronasal breathing.

In a study of pediatric patients whose oronasal breathing and elevated nasal resistances had been quantitatively assessed, the nasal fraction of respiratory airflow increased on reduction of nasal resistance by means of topical decongestant.[52] Although it seems reasonable to expect, and there is evidence to suggest, that the nasal fraction increases together with patency as subjects age,[105, 106] analysis of our own results from 120 children have not supported this view.

In contrast to the increased nasal fraction of oronasal airflow resulting from increased nasal patency in children, and, as might be expected, the reverse was found to accompany artificial increases in nasal resistance during voluntary oronasal breathing in healthy adult volunteers.[52, 53]

It appears that in oronasal breathing the degree of nasal patency plays a part in distribution of respiratory air between nose and mouth. But the mouth provides a far greater range of airflow resistances than the nose, and the variable cross section of the labial aperture is the major determinant of oral airflow resistance and resulting oronasal distribution of respiratory airflow.

Parapalatal Airways

The soft palate can occlude either the oral or the nasal airway, and its intermediate positioning between tongue and posterior pharyngeal wall enables oronasal breathing to take place.[82] In awake, healthy subjects breathing exclusively through the nose, determinations of respiratory airflow resistances above and below the soft palate have been made. They have shown resistance of the palatopharyngeal airway segment to be small during the posterior rhinomanometric maneuver (Chapter 4) by comparison with resistance of either the oral or nasal vestibules.[11, 41] Furthermore, these resistances were reported to be unaffected by retraction of the soft palate with a suture through the uvula.[99] As already mentioned, the palatoglossal segment of the airways presents similarly small resistance to airflow during oral breathing.[9] Thus, the principal resistors affecting oronasal breathing and its distribution are situated at the oral and nasal portals rather than the parapalatal airways.

In the panting dog, however, cineradiography has shown the soft palate to be the principal structural component regulating the path of respiratory airflow.[2] It directs ambient inspiratory air through the nose and warm, moist expiratory air through the mouth.[87] Shallow breathing shunts dead-space air to and fro, maximizing heat loss and minimizing disturbance of alveolar carbon dioxide and acid-base balance.

The spontaneous pursed-lip mode of breathing adopted during physical effort by patients suffering from chronic obstructive pulmonary disease includes closure of the palatopharyngeal aperture.[83] Palatal occlusion is required also in articulation, swallowing, sneezing, whistling, puffing, blowing, and in the Müeller and Valsalva and other breathing maneuvers.[82] In many of these activities pursing of the lips is accompanied by adduction of the vocal cords (N. Zamel, personal communication, 1991). The soft palate appears to function more as an on/off switch than as a variable resistor in awake human subjects.

THE THROAT

The Pharyngeal Airway

The pharynx is necessarily a compliant and muscular passage with few skeletal restrictions. It enables brief acts of swallowing to convey material from the mouth and from the mucociliary transport system of the air passages to the esophagus. Apart from these momentary swallowing interruptions, the pharynx must provide an adequate respiratory airway.

Neuromuscular coordination between pharyngeal and laryngeal dilators and constrictors is essential for control of swallowing and breathing. Dysfunction can have disastrous consequences at this critical intersection of swallowing and breathing passages, since diversion of solids and liquids from the airway and continuous pulmonary ventilation are essential for life. Impaired consciousness from any cause (sedative drugs, anesthesia, head injury, sleep, etc.) threatens patency of the upper airway and its respiratory function.[34]

Twenty-four upper-airway muscles (including six intrinsic to the larynx) affect compliance, caliber resistance, and flow limitation of this region.[78] These muscles can maximize or occlude the airway, and several have additional functions that differ from the respiratory role they are recruited to perform. Their phasic respiratory dilating and stabilizing actions are somewhat analogous to those of the intercostals[78] with which they are normally coordinated.

The U-shaped cartilages of the trachea, with their posterior musculature, have skeletal analogs in the thyroid, hyoid, mandibular, and skull-base structures that provide attachments for lumen-modifying muscles of the pharynx.[110] Apart from brief intervals of swallowing, muscles attached to the skull base, mandible, and sternum play an essential part in restraining compliance of neck and pharyngeal tissues with gravity and inspiratory transmural pressures, thus contributing to preservation of a patent pharyngeal lumen. Electromyographic studies have shown phasic increase in inspiratory activity of airway dilator muscles in humans and animals during spontaneous breathing—and further increase upon elevation of airway resistance. In addition, studies indicate that the tone of these airway dilating muscles increases in response to subatmospheric airway pressures in animals,[56] and in humans to increases in nasal resistance.[111]

The Unconscious Pharynx

As already described, in healthy, awake subjects the palatoglossal and palatopharyngeal segments present relatively small resistances to respiratory airflow, and the soft palate provides a switching mechanism that can occlude either airway or leave both patent. In sleep and other forms of diminished consciousness, upper-airway dilator muscle tone is diminished also, and under these circumstances, flaccidity of the tissues and gravitational forces combine to narrow the parapalatal and glossopharyngeal airways (Fig 2–2). Further narrowing is promoted by compliance with the subatmospheric pressures that are generated within the pharyngeal lumen by inspiration against upstream resistances.

Constriction of the airway induces airflow conditions that tend to promote further constriction. As linear velocity of the narrowed pharyngeal airstream is increased, in order to maintain the flow necessary for pulmonary ventilation, transmural differential pressures are increased further at the site of narrowing (Bernoulli), thereby contributing to the summation of forces tending to promote occlusion of the pharyngeal lumen.

Narrowing increases resistance to airflow, and, indeed, it has been noted that pharyngeal respiratory airflow resistance is elevated in apneic patients.[1] Airway constriction may lead to partial obstruction of sufficient severity to induce noisy breathing, snoring, or both; this occurs at lesser transmural differential pressures in chronic snorers and apneic patients than in subjects in whom these obstructive events are not manifested spontaneously.[39, 40] Noisy breathing and snores result from a Starling valve effect of flaccid pharyngeal and surrounding cervical tissues.

Furthermore, if a critical inspiratory transmural pressure is achieved, the pharyngeal walls collapse completely and occlude the airway (see Figs 2–2 and 2–3). As the closing pressure occludes the pharyngeal lumen,

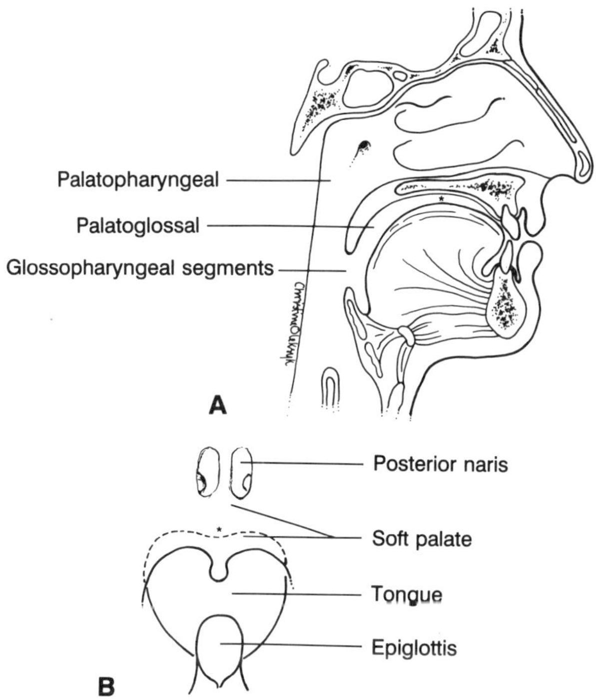

FIG 2–2.

The parapalatal (palatoglossal and palatopharyngeal) airways. **A,** sagittal section of upper airways. **B,** Anterior pharynx from behind.

inspiratory efforts increase transmural pressures further and seal the closure more tightly, resulting in an obstructive apnea that is maintained until arousal reactivates dilator muscle tone and restores airway patency. Subatmospheric esophageal pressures reflect those in the pharynx below an apneic obstruction.[101] Pressures >60 cms H_2O below atmospheric have been recorded.

Measurements by inductive plethysmography show a reduced inspiratory cross-sectional area of the neck to accompany snoring, apneas, and hypopneas, and the area is increased in expiration. In labored breathing, cross-sectional areas of chest and neck are 180° out of phase.[55]

In sleep, pharyngeal resistances peak as airflow velocities peak during inspiration and reach high values even in healthy nonsnoring male subjects with normal nasal resistances.[37] Also, in healthy sleeping subjects, pharyngeal inspiratory resistances are reduced when nasal resistances are decreased by topical decongestant. These pharyngeal resistances are increased not only by sleep but also by dorsal recumbency.[1, 35]

Obstructive Apneas

As already described, the resistive behavior of the pharynx in sleeping subjects indicates narrowing in compliance with inspiratory transmural pressures. The principal sites of narrowing and increased resistance have been identified as the palatopharyngeal and glossopharyngeal segments of the airway in healthy subjects and, in patients, apneic obstructions have been demonstrated at these same two sites (Fig 2–3). In the majority of apneic patients, obstruction occurs at the palatal level,[7, 36, 62–64] but the site of occlusion is not predictable from measurements in awake subjects.

Passavant's bar, a prominent muscular ridge that can be seen occupying the palatopharyngeal aperture posteriorly in patients with cleft palate, may play a part also in apneic occlusions. Furthermore, it should be noted that

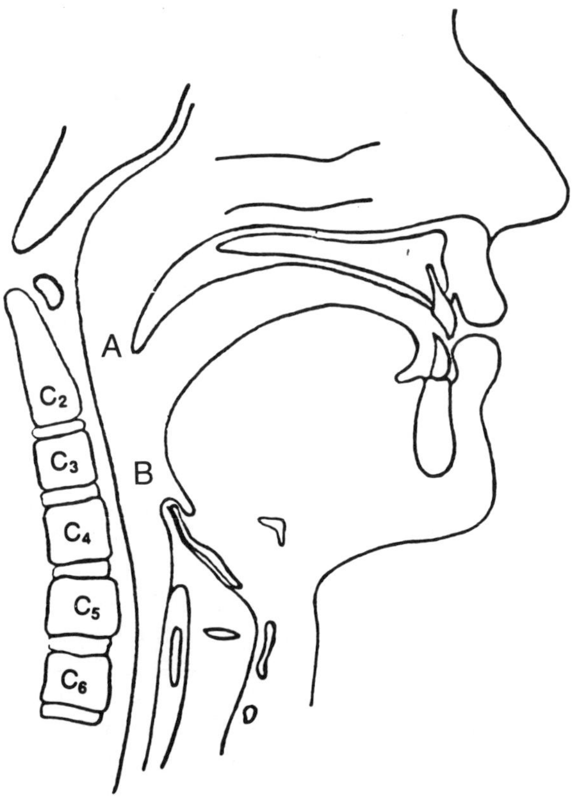

FIG 2–3.

Sites and incidence of obstruction in 37 cases of obstructive apnea syndrome. **A,** greater than two thirds; **B,** less than one third.

apneic palatopharyngeal closure may have preceded or accompanied the glossopharyngeal closures that were registered by our catheter studies of pharyngeal pressures.[7] It is possible that the palatopharynx is the primary site of obstruction and closure of the glossopharyngeal segment is secondary to it.

Snoring, other obstructive events, and interrupted sleep may be exacerbated by elevated upstream nasal resistances that increase inspiratory pharyngeal transmural pressures[21] and are reflected in intra-esophageal pressure swings.[74, 75, 101] Similarly, nasal obstructions resulting from seasonal attacks of allergic rhinitis and from septal deviations have been reported to impair sleep quality and to increase the frequency and duration of apneas. These manifestations are relieved by successful nasal therapy or by spontaneous resolution of the provoking condition.[48–50, 59, 116]

Artificially induced subatmospheric airway pressures provoke obstructive apneas in sleeping subjects and increased pharyngeal resistance in awake apneics.[88, 95] Conversely, pressures greater than atmospheric (10 to 15 cm H_2O), applied also via a nasal mask, splint the pharynx and abolish both snoring and obstructive incidents in apneic patients. This latter technique is employed therapeutically in sleeping apneic patients as *continuous positive airway pressure (CPAP).*[94]

Both central and obstructive apneas and disordered breathing can be induced in healthy sleeping subjects by application of a topical anesthetic to the pharynx and to the normally patent nose. The obstructive responses are of similar magnitude to those obtained by nasal occlusion, suggesting that fifth-nerve and, possibly, pharyngeal sensory nerve stimulation may play an important part in breathing and upper-airway patency[58, 60, 86, 109] (see Chapter 4, "Symptomatology").

SNORING

More Than a Joke

Despite its comic aspects, snoring has serious pathologic and sociologic repercussions. Epidemiological studies indicate that it is a risk factor in many diseases[72] (Table 2–1), and it is a universal accompaniment of obstructive sleep apnea syndrome.

Sociologic impacts of snoring include family discord, deterrence or dissolution of friendships and marriages, and even murders have been reported.[15] Snores with a sound intensity level that is regarded as hazardous in an industrial setting have been reported and yet do not wake the snorer. Recordings of 90 db snores were obtained from a 40-year-old male subject

TABLE 2–1.
Medical Problems and Snoring*†

Condition	All	Non-snorers	Occasional Snorers	Those Who Snore Nearly Every Night	Those Who Snore Every Night
Overweight	7•2	2•3	8•9	16•9	22•8
Smoker†	17•9	10•3	24•0	32•9	33•9
Raised blood pressure†	6•2	2•3	8•8	12•2	18•5
Insomnia	1•3	0•6	1•7	5•6	1•6
Chest disease†	2•2	1•4	2•7	4•7	5•1
Heart disease†	4•2	1•7	5•5	9•9	11•8
Depression†	0•8	0•2	1•3	2•8	2•0
Alcoholism†	0•5		0•2	2•3	2•0
Diabetes†	1•5	0•8	2•0	2•3	3•5
Sleep during day†	1•3	0•2	2•0	4•7	3•2
Rheumatism†	4•4	2•1	7•1	8•5	9•1
Allergies†	11•2	9•6	13•8	14•1	14•2
Asthma	2•9	2•0	5•0	3•8	2•0
Other†	7•3	4•6	8•9	11•7	15•0
Total No. in each group	2,629	1,379	638	213	254
Men (%)	53•7	45•4	64•2	69•0	73•2
Husbands (%)	20•9	11•7	34•9	41•8	37•8

*From Norton PG, Dunn EV: Snoring as a risk factor for disease: An epidemiological survey. *Br Med J* 1985; 291:630. Used by permission.
†Values are percentages.
‡$p < 0 \cdot 001$, χ^2 test for trend; all tests for linearity NS.

at the Department of Medicine, University of British Columbia.[23] Innocent victims live in dread of nightly torment of which their torturer remains blissfully unaware. However, victims are avenged in some cases by the course of nature and the grave consequences of obstructed breathing that befall the snorer.

At least one snorer lurks in 80% of households. In a recent survey regular snoring was reported in 86% of married men and 57% of their wives; while 56% of women were bothered by snoring of a spouse, only 15% of men had this complaint.[71] Zoo studies have revealed that many different animals snore, too. Uveopalatopharyngoplasty (UPPP), as performed for relief of snoring in humans, is a well-recognized therapeutic measure for this disease in bulldogs.

Snoring indicates partial airway obstruction.[74] It is brought about by interaction between kinetic energy of the respiratory airstream ($E = k\dot{V}^2$) and the flaccid soft palate and flabby tissues surrounding the parapalatal airways. It is an indication of airway narrowing. The resulting increased linear velocity of the narrowed airstream and a Starling valve effect produce fluttering vibrations that are in the audible frequency range. Snores can be generated by nose or mouth breathing and by inspiration or expiration. The most formidable snores, however, are produced by nasal inspirations, and they may be amplified by resonance in an open mouth.

Snoring can be regarded as a breathing disorder of sleep, one that, although it indicates partial airway obstruction, is so commonplace and so apparently benign that in the majority of cases it can be regarded as a relatively harmless respiratory aberration from a pathologic (if not sociologic) point of view. Nevertheless, a patient with the complaint of snoring deserves to be taken seriously, for a careful history and examination may reveal important underlying pathology. As already emphasized, heavy snoring is a consistent accompaniment of obstructive sleep apnea syndrome.

Although an association between elevated nasal resistance and snoring is widely accepted, the relationship is inconstant; indeed, our rhinomanometric experience with several hundred snorers while they were awake has not shown marked elevation to be a predominant feature.

Nocturnal polysomnography, which includes recording of frequency, duration, and intensity of snoring, is performed in patients referred to our sleep laboratory at St. Michael's Hospital, Toronto, for investigation of the complaint of heavy snoring and suspected sleep apnea syndrome.[31, 30] Rhinomanometry is performed on these patients in the awake state and seated posture, not concomitantly with the sleep study. A positive correlation between snoring and body mass index has been found,[62–64] with no significant differences in snoring between sexes (77 females and 293 males were studied) or between apneics and non-apneics. Retrospective analysis of variance of data from 683 patients showed no significant differences of apnea or snoring indices among three groups of patients—one group with normal, another with elevated unilateral, and a third with elevated bilateral nasal resistances.[65]

The above nasal resistance measurements that were made in awake, seated subjects may not have been representative of the situation in sleep. Indeed, it is probable that there were cases where resistances were amplified in recumbency by nasal mucovascular dysfunction or structural abnormality (see Chapter 1). However, a current study of resistance measurements of healthy noses in eight snoring patients, taken during sleep, has shown no significant correlation between nasal patency and snoring to date.

Although subatmospheric inspiratory pressures can narrow the pharyngeal airway in sleeping subjects, therapeutic results of decreasing upstream resistances by stenting the nasal valve (see Chapter 1, "Nasal Valve") and by topical decongestant have been disappointing.[3] Recordings of intensity, frequency, and duration of heavy snoring were unaffected by substantial reduction of nasal resistance by stenting in all four stages of sleep and oxygen desaturation were not relieved.[64] In another series of investigations, stenting in combination with topical decongestant resulted in a striking increase in nasal patency but failed to reduce the apnea index in patients with obstructive sleep apnea syndrome.[44]

It has been suggested that nasal resistance may be influenced also by sleep stages that alter both autonomic and alar dilator muscle activity, but our study of postnasal pressure recordings of respiratory airflow obtained from 32 sleeping subjects did not support this view (Cole and Lavie, unpublished, 1984).

There seems little doubt that severe nasal obstruction leads to breathing disorders in sleep,[74] but the relative importance of lesser degrees of obstruction or their relief has not been clearly demonstrated (see also the next section in this chapter, under the subhead of "Treatment of Obstructive Breathing in Sleep").

SLEEP APNEA SYNDROME

A Serious Disease

Since the 1970s[89] the clinical importance of breathing disorders in sleep has been well established, and a complex of symptoms and signs in which apneas predominate has become widely recognized as a distinct clinical entity (Fig 2–4). Clinicians are alerted by complaints of a patient's snoring and apneic incidents that may indicate a potentially lethal disease,[27, 77] and these

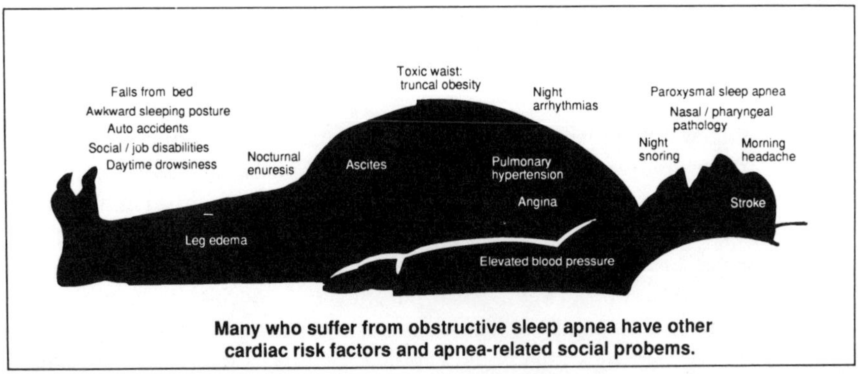

FIG 2–4.

Profile typifies a patient with idiopathic obstructive apnea. (From Swift D: Sleep apnea, heart disease, double cardiac death risk. *Med Post* 1991; Jan 15:13. Used by permission.)

manifestations in obese, male patients who complain also of excessive daytime sleepiness sharpen the index of suspicion.[80] Snoring, apneas, and the signs and symptoms that result from sleep fragmentation and repeated hypoxemia may not be evident to the patient, and history obtained from a close associate often plays an important part in diagnosis.

Obstructive sleep apnea syndrome is nowadays encountered on a weekly basis by many family practitioners,[22, 45] and lay public awareness of the symptoms and implications of the disease has increased concomitantly with that of the medical profession. In such patients consideration should be given to diagnostic sleep monitoring, especially if, in addition to snoring and apneas, there is a suggestion of excessive daytime sleepiness.[54]

Sleep Laboratories

In the course of the last decade "sleep medicine" has gained increasing recognition as a subspecialty. Consequently, appropriately equipped facilities for diagnosing and treating sleep disorders have been established in many urban centers of the Western world. Obstructive sleep apnea is the most common sleep disorder investigated in these centers. Specialized professionals there attempt to determine the severity of the condition and the need for intervention. The syndrome is not confined to adults. In fact, early reports concerned children with hypertrophied adenoid and/or tonsil obstruction[14] and associated cor pulmonale.[57] And Charles Dickens's description of the "Pickwickian syndrome" is legendary.

Significant breathing disorders in sleep have been estimated to adversely affect 1% to 2% of an adult working population[47] and >2% of the general white population.[22] These disorders are positively correlated with work accidents, absenteeism, and an increase in cardiovascular morbidity and mortality risk.

Clinical Presentation

Obstructive breathing in sleep presents as a continuum that extends from snoring without evidence of serious pathologic sequelae to repeated apneas and hypopneas with severe oxygen desaturation, sleep fragmentation, and attendant complications. Progression toward the more severely obstructive phase is promoted by depression of the nervous system by alcohol, sedative drugs, or disease; by excessive body mass; and by structural obstructions of the supraglottic airways. Histologic changes associated with snoring have been found in the pharyngeal mucosa, but they could be results of vibratory trauma rather than the cause of snoring.[91]

Idiopathic obstructive sleep apnea syndrome is predominantly a male disease, probably dependent on a genetic predisposition and worsened by excess body mass.[47] It is uncertain whether the underlying airway instability is neurologic or morphologic.

Although the disease is predominantly a male disorder, breathing and oxygenation during sleep are similar in healthy men and women. Furthermore, apneic and hypopneic events are common and symptomless in both sexes; they increase in frequency with age and do not necessarily imply an unfavorable prognosis.[6] The frequency of apneic incidents is increased in "mouth breathers," and mouth breathing is more common in men than women. This tendency, too, is increased in sleeping subjects and with age.[20]

Frequency of apneic and hypopneic incidents correlates significantly not only with body-mass index but with external neck circumference. This suggests the possibility that pharyngeal size is modulated by dynamic loading from weight of fatty cervical tissue,[43] but in our limited experience, cervical liposuction has not reduced the incidence of pathologic pharyngeal obstructions.

Upper-airway obstruction in sleeping subjects can lead to the hypoventilation that plays an important part in the pathogenesis of hypertension, cardiac arrhythmias, and cardiac insufficiency, and shortens life expectancy of the middle aged.[77] An extensive catalog of pathologic consequences associated with obstructive sleep apnea syndrome exists. Some are listed in Table 2–2 and illustrated in Fig 2–4.

Clinical Assessment of Sleep Apnea Syndrome

Universal agreement is lacking not only as to a precise definition of sleep apnea syndrome but also as to the prognostic significance of the clinical

TABLE 2–2.
Pathologic Consequences of Obstructive Sleep Apnea Syndrome

Neuropsychologic	Cardiovascular
Hypersomnolence	Elevated catecholamine
Impaired memory	Systemic hypertension
Impaired concentration	Pulmonary hypertension
Mood and personality change	Cardiac arrhythmias
Depression	Cardiac failure
Psychosis	Cardiac death
Impotence	
Inattention	
Accident proneness	
Nocturnal enuresis	

findings. Frequency of obstructive incidents is highly variable from night to night if apneas number <100/night, but are more consistent when this number is exceeded.[112] The overlap between normal and pathologic breathing in sleep is wide, and as mentioned earlier, neither snoring nor apneas are uncommon in apparently healthy subjects.

In less severe cases, prognosis is less predictable and the appropriateness of available forms of management is not firmly established. But severe obstructive sleep apnea leads to morbidity and death and leaves little doubt as to the urgency for treatment. It is important, therefore, that an accurate diagnosis and assessment of severity of suspected sleep apnea syndrome be consolidated by sleep studies.

Diagnosis of Obstructive Sleep Apnea Syndrome

A practical series of requirements that satisfy a diagnosis of sleep apnea syndrome includes ten or more incidents of apnea or hypopnea per hour, each of 10 seconds duration or longer and accompanied by oxygen desaturation of 4% or more. Hypopnea is defined as 50% or greater reduction in tidal volume. The diagnosis is commonly substantiated by findings of heavy snoring, excessive daytime sleepiness, and headache or nausea on waking. Additional signs, symptoms, and complications are listed in Table 2–2.

Apneas are termed *obstructive* when accompanied by respiratory efforts and *central* when no respiratory efforts are made. The patients referred for investigation in sleep laboratories are most commonly in the obstructive category. Obstructive apneas can be secondary to structural abnormalities such as micrognathia, hyperglossia, or tonsil or adenoid hypertrophy, but in the majority of adult patients the condition is idiopathic.

Diagnostic data can be acquired by home monitoring equipment, but at the present time most North American patients with suspected breathing disorders of sleep are investigated in sleep laboratories. Signals obtained by sensors applied to the patient are registered by a polygraph strip chart recorder as the patient sleeps. The following investigations are common to most sleep laboratories:

1. Electroencephalography to determine sleep stage
2. Electro-oculography to detect REM sleep
3. Electromyography to monitor pharyngeal dilator muscle activity (genioglossus)
4. Electrocardiography to detect cardiac irregularities
5. Testing of thoracic and abdominal breathing movements
6. Testing of nasal and oral airflow

7. Skin-surface oximetry (ear or finger) to determine oxygen saturation

Additional investigations are performed according to the interests and preferences of the investigators. In awake patients, the following may be performed:

1. Pulmonary function tests
2. Measurement of nasal airflow resistance[7, 62–64]
3. Testing of pharyngeal acoustic reflection[18, 33]
4. Lateral cephalic and other X-ray examinations
5. Measurement of body mass index

In awake or sleeping patients, the following may be performed:

1. Cineradiography of the pharynx
2. Computed tomography[24, 96]
3. Measurement of snoring frequency, duration, and intensity
4. Measurement of nasal airflow resistance
5. Sonography of breathing sounds
6. Recording of limb movements during sleep
7. Video recording of sleeping patients
8. Measurement of pharyngeal respiratory airflow pressures[62–64]
9. Inductive plethysmographic recording of abdominal and thoracic breathing
10. Pernasal fiber-optic pharyngoscopy
11. Somnofluoroscopy[42]

The inductive plethysmographic technique, which determines volume change of a cylinder from changes in its circumference, is minimally invasive and has been used to measure changes in cervical cross section[55] and to measure and record respiratory volume changes of the thorax and abdomen.[107]

Lateral cephalic X-ray examination is employed for soft-tissue assessment to determine dimensions of the pharyngeal airway and obstructive potential of adenoid and tonsil hypertrophy, bulky tongue, soft palate and/or uvula, and for measurements between bony landmarks to estimate the normality of skeletal proportions. Opinions differ as to the diagnostic value of computed tomography (CT)[24] and fluoroscopy in awake apneic patients. Abnormal pharyngeal dimensions were not evident in a series of CT scans of awake, obese apneic patients who showed elevated upper-airway resistance to breathing.[90] Somnofluoroscopy is reported to reveal pharyngeal narrowing in apneic patients either above or below the midpoint of vertebra C2, the upper level indicating probability of a favorable result from UPPP.[42]

The latter findings are contrary to our own experience in patients with moderately severe obstructive disease.[62–64] UPPP was successful in reducing obstructive events and snoring in only a minority of these patients, and results were no better in patients with demonstrated obstruction at palatal level than in those with obstruction in the glossopharynx.

Clinical comment. Breathing disorders in sleep are common and often benign, but in some cases they can cause morbidity and threaten life. Sleep studies are essential for diagnosis, for assessment of severity, and for therapeutic guidance.

Treatment of Obstructive Breathing in Sleep

If findings are judged to indicate a significant risk factor, many therapeutic options are available[4] depending on the severity of the findings. The following therapeutic measures are usually applied in combination or in a stepwise manner.

1. Weight control
2. Sedative and alcohol limitation
3. Correction of anatomic abnormalities
4. Adenotonsillectomy
5. Treatment of nasal obstruction
6. Continuous positive airway pressure (CPAP)[93, 94]
7. Uveopalatopharyngoplasty (UPPP)[19, 62–64]
8. Gastric stapling
9. Cervical liposuction
10. Reduction glossoplasty[19]
11. Skeletal advancements of hyoid, mandible, and/or maxilla[79]
12. Tracheostomy

Drug treatments and oral prostheses have not established a successful record. Patient tolerance and patient compliance limit the value of several effective treatment modalities such as weight control, sedative restriction, and nasopharyngeal intubation.

Although some therapeutic measures may appear rather drastic, they are justified by serious morbidity and lethal potential of severe obstructive sleep apnea syndrome. Application of CPAP to sleeping patients splints the pharynx, and tracheostomy bypasses the pharynx; each completely relieves snoring and idiopathic obstructive sleep apnea syndrome. Either method may be successful in controlling the condition and improving prognosis, but there are patients for whom neither is acceptable.[13]

UPPP is an alternative for such patients. However, in many centers, objective assessments have shown results of UPPP alone to be unpredictable,[19, 62–64, 115] so this procedure is increasingly employed in conjunction with other surgical measures such as glossoplasty or skeletal advancements.

An adverse relationship between nasal obstruction and breathing in sleep appears well established, and there are numerous anecdotal reports that relief of nasal obstruction is accompanied by relief of sleep breathing disorders.[15] This latter view is supported by objective evidence of the beneficial effects of both spontaneous relief and of therapy of nasal obstruction on the quality of sleep and on sleep breathing disorders.[49, 50] However, substantial acute increases in nasal patency during sleep by stenting the nasal valve and applying topical decongestant over a single night have proved less successful on objective assessment (as discussed previously). It is possible that the more optimistic anecdotal and subjective reports result from longer duration than overnight of the effects of therapeutic or spontaneous resolution of nasal obstruction.

Objective patency and snoring assessments in addition to routine polysomnography are required before and after nasal therapy to clarify relationships between nasal patency and breathing in sleep and to resolve the apparent discrepancy between anecdotal and objective findings. Universal standards for therapeutic success have not been established, and reported success rates vary widely. Stringent criteria lower apparent success markedly. Few long-term results have been published.[12]

It is not unusual for objective sleep studies to fail in detecting improvement while subjective reports by patients and other observers surpass expectations.[108] Complaints of excessive daytime sleepiness and snoring fall into this category. Although analysis of the results of many surgical measures is inconclusive, there seems little doubt as to the effectiveness of either tracheostomy or CPAP on signs, symptoms, and prognosis.[76]

It has been suggested that the pharyngeal airway is in the final common path of a more widely or remotely situated disease that might explain the success of splinting or bypassing the pharynx and the unpredictability of results of local surgical treatments.[32]

Risk Factors and Interventions

As mentioned above, in the present state of clinical knowledge and experience, risk factors and appropriate interventions are not firmly established for moderate degrees of obstructive apnea, but an apnea index of <7 has been shown to be an independent risk factor in cardiac attacks,[38] and there are many other situations where consideration of intervention is warranted. Heavy snoring may be a severe social handicap or herald domestic disaster and justify treatment for that reason. Operation of machinery (e.g., an automobile)[16] by an apneic patient with excessive daytime sleepiness is an accident waiting to happen. The danger to patients themselves and to family members, colleagues, and strangers presents a compelling reason for intervention. There are many less dramatic psychiatric sequelae and hypersomnic disabilities that affect employment, scholastic, and social activities of both adults and children and thus demand at least consideration of the need for clinical interference. These disabilities may be unrecognized by the patient but reported by an observant relative or close associate.

A medical practitioner must take into account a wide range of diagnostic, prognostic, and therapeutic considerations when faced with the problems of patients whose symptoms suggest the possibility of obstructed breathing in sleep. Continued accumulation and analysis of reliable data should provide increasing guidance for appropriate management of this relatively newly recognized clinical entity.

SUMMARY

In awake subjects the mouth provides an alternative respiratory airway to the nose. When lips and mandible are spontaneously positioned, it is a resistor of similar magnitude to the nasal valve. The mouth is effective also as a conditioner and cleanser of inspiratory air (see Chapter 3), but, unlike the nose, the mouth requires frequent remoistening with saliva. Exclusive oral breathing is exceptional, and oronasal breathing in awake subjects is pathologic only when it is chronic; but neither the chronically open mouth nor partial nasal obstruction furnish a reliable clinical guide to the existence or extent of mouth breathing. Objective assessment is a valuable aid to diagnosis and a guide to management (see Chapter 4). It provides impartial follow-up and indispensable research data.

Definitive relationships between dentofacial morphology and nasal- and oral-airway function have not been established with certainty, but in view of the credible risks of developmental abnormalities that are unlikely to resolve spontaneously, lengthy expectant treatment of chronic upper-airway obstruction is seldom justified. Although nasal and other upper-airway obstructions can lead to significant breathing disorders in sleep, these consequences are not yet universally recognized, nor are therapeutic results firmly established by objective testing.

Soft-tissue or skeletal disproportion, elevated upstream resistance, or neuromuscular dysfunction all promote pharyngeal compliance and narrowing in sleeping subjects, resulting in partial obstruction of respiratory airflow, snoring, and apneas. Patency of the oral airway is unreliable in sleep, so nasal patency assumes increased importance.

Snoring and apneas are common in healthy men and women, but significant breathing disorders of sleep affect >2% of Caucasian populations. Pathologic obstructive sleep apneas are associated with the male sex, obesity, and central nervous system depression, and the majority of adult cases are idiopathic. Since obstructive sleep apnea syndrome is a source of morbidity, and it can be lethal, accurate diagnosis by sleep studies and other measures is essential. Effective therapies are available.

REFERENCES

1. Anch AM, Remmers JE, Bunce H III: Supraglottic airway resistance in normal subjects and patients with occlusive sleep apnea. *J Appl Physiol* 1982; 53(5):1158–1163.
2. Biewener AA, Soghikian GW, Crompton AW: Regulation and respiratory airflow during panting and feeding in the dog. *Resp Physiol* 1985; 61:185–195.
3. Blakely BW, Mahowald MW: Nasal resistance and sleep apnea. *Laryngoscope* 1987; 97:752–754.
4. Bradley D, Phillipson EA: The treatment of obstructive sleep apnea: separating the wheat from the chaff. *Am Rev Respir Dis* 1983; 128:583–586.
5. Camner P, Bakke B: Nose or mouth breathing? *Environ Res* 1980; 21:394–398.
6. Catterall JR, Calverley PMA, Shapiro CM, et al: Breathing and oxygenation during sleep are similar in normal men and women. *Am Rev Respir Dis* 1985; 132:86–88.
7. Chaban R, Cole P, Hoffstein V: Site of upper airway obstruction in patients with idiopathic obstructive sleep apnea. *Laryngoscope* 1988; 98:641–647.
8. Chada TS, Birch S, Sacker MA: Oronasal distribution of ventilation during exercise in normal subjects and patients with asthma and rhinitis. *Chest* 1987; 92(6):1037–1041.
9. Cole P, Forsyth R, Haight JSJ: Respiratory resistance of the oral airway. *Am Rev Respir Dis* 1982; 125:363–365.
10. Cole P, Naito K, Chaban R, et al: Unilateral and bilateral nasal resistance. *Rhinology* 1988; 26:209–216.
11. Cole P, Ayiomamitis A, Ohki M. Anterior and posterior rhinomanometry. *Rhinology* 1989; 27:257–262.
12. Conway WA, Fujita S, Zorick F, et al: Uvulopalatopharyngoplasty. One-year followup. *Chest* 1985; 88:385–387.
13. Conway WA, Victor LD, Magilligan DJ, et al: Adverse effects of tracheostomy for sleep apnea. *JAMA* 1981; 246:347–350.
14. Croft CB, Brockbank MJ, Wright A, et al: Obstructive sleep apnoea in chil-

dren undergoing routine tonsillectomy and adenoidectomy. *Clin Otolaryngol* 1990; 15:307–314.
15. Fairbanks DNF: Effect of nasal surgery on snoring. *South Med J* 1985; 78:268–270.
16. Findley LJ, Unverzagt ME, Suratt PM: Automobile accidents involving patients with obstructive sleep apnea. *Am Rev Respir Dis* 1988; 138(2):337–340.
17. Forsyth RD, Cole P, Shephard RJ: Exercise and nasal patency. *J Appl Physiol* 1983; 55(3):860–865.
18. Fredberg JJ, Wohl MV, Glass GM, et al: Airway area by acoustic reflections measured at the mouth. *J Appl Physiol* 1980; 48:749–758.
19. Fujita S: Surgical treatment of obstructive sleep apnea: UPPP and linguoplasty (laser mid-line glossectomy), in Guilleminault C, Partinen M (eds): *Obstructive Sleep Apnea Syndrome: Clinical Research and Treatment.* New York, Raven Press, 1990.
20. Gleeson K, Zwillich CW, Braier K, et al: Breathing route during sleep. *Am Rev Respir Dis* 1966; 134:115–120.
21. Gleeson K, Zwillich CW, Bendrick TW, et al: Effect of inspiratory nasal loading on pharyngeal resistance. *J Appl Physiol* 1986; 60(6):1882–1886.
22. Guilleminault C, Partinen M: Preface, in Guilleminault C, Partinen M (eds): *Obstructive Sleep Apnea Syndrome: Clinical Research and Treatment.* New York, Raven Press, 1987.
23. *Guinness Book of Records 1990.* United Kingdom, Guinness Publishing Co., 1991, p 18.
24. Haponik EF, Smith PL, Bohlman ME, et al: Computerized tomography in obstructive sleep apnea. Correlation of airway size with physiology during sleep and wakefulness. *Am Rev Respir Dis* 1983; 127.221–226.
25. Harvold EP, Tomer BS, Vargervik K, et al: Primate experiments on oral respiration. *Am J Orthod* 1981; 79(4):359–372.
26. Harvold EP, Vargervik K: Experiments on the interaction between orofacial function and morphology. *Ear Nose Throat J* 1987; 66:26–39.
27. He J, Kryger MH, Conway WA, et al: Mortality and apnea index in obstructive sleep apnea. *Chest* 1988; 94:9–14.
28. Hinton VA, Warren DW, Hairfield WM: Upper airway pressures during breathing: A comparison of normal and nasally incompetent subjects with modeling studies. *Am J Orthod* 1986; 89(6):492–498.
29. Hinton VA, Warren DW, Hairfield WM, et al: The relationship between nasal cross-sectional area and nasal air volume in normal and nasally impaired adults. *Am J Orthod Dentofacial Orthop* 1987; 92:294–298.
30. Hoffstein V, Meteike JH, Mateika S: Snoring and sleep architecture. *Am Rev Respir Dis* 1991; 143:92–96.
31. Hoffstein V, Chaban R, Cole P, et al: Snoring and upper airway properties. *Chest* 1988; 94:87–89.
32. Hoffstein V, Zamel N: Sleep apnea and the upper airway. *Br J Anaesth* 1990; 65:139–150.
33. Hoffstein V, Fredberg JJ: The acoustic reflection technique for non-invasive assessment of upper airway area. *Eur Respir J* 1991 (in press).

34. Horner RL, Guz A: Some factors affecting maintenance of upper airway patency in man. *Respir Med* 1991; 85(suppl A):27–30.
35. Hudgel DW, Robertson DW: Nasal resistance during wakefulness and sleep in normal man. *Acta Otolaryngol (Stockh)* 1984; 98:130–135.
36. Hudgel DW: Variable site of narrowing among obstructive sleep apnea patients. *J Appl Physiol* 1986; 61(4):1403–1409.
37. Hudgel DW, Hendricks C: Palate and hypopharynx: Sites of inspiratory narrowing of the upper airway during sleep. *Am Rev Respir Dis* 1988; 138:1542–1547.
38. Hung J, Whitford EG, Parsons RW, et al: Association of sleep apnea with myocardial infarction in men. *Lancet* 1990; 336:261–264.
39. Issa FG, Sullivan CE: Upper airway closing pressures in obstructive sleep apnea. *J Appl Physiol* 1984; 57:520–527.
40. Issa FG, Sullivan CE: Upper airway pressure in snorers. *J Appl Physiol* 1984; 57:528–535.
41. Jones AS, Lancer JM, Stevens JC, et al: Rhinomanometry: Do the anterior and posterior methods give equivalent results? *Clin Otolaryngol* 1987; 12:109–114.
42. Katsantonis GP, Walsh JK: Somnofluoroscopy: its role in the selection of candidates for uvulopalatopharyngoplasty. *Otolaryngol Head Neck Surg* 1986; 94(1):56–60.
43. Katz I, Stradling J, Slutsky AS, et al: Do patients with obstructive sleep apnea have thick necks? *Am Rev Respir Dis* 1990; 141:1228–1231.
44. Kerr P, Kryger M, Miller T, et al: The importance of nasal airflow resistance in obstructive sleep apnea syndrome. *J Otolaryngol* 1991(suppl 1); 20:25.
45. Kimoff RJ, Cosio MG, McGregor M: Clinical features and treatment of obstructive sleep apnea. *Can Med Assoc J* 1991; 144(6): 689–695.
46. Klein JC: Nasal respiratory function and craniofacial growth. *Arch Otolaryngol Head Neck Surg* 1986; 112:843–849.
47. Lavie P: Incidence of sleep apnea in a presumably healthy working population: A significant relationship with excessive daytime sleepiness. *Sleep* 1983; 6(4):312–318.
48. Lavie P, Fischel N, Zomer J, et al: The effects of partial and complete mechanical occlusion of the nasal passages on sleep structure and breathing in sleep. *Acta Otolaryngol (Stockh)* 1983; 95:161–166.
49. Lavie P, Gertner R, Zomer J, et al: Breathing disorders in sleep associated with microarousals in patients with allergic rhinitis. *Acta Otolaryngol (Stockh)* 1981; 92:529–533.
50. Lavie P, Zomer J, Eliaschar I, et al: Excessive daytime sleepiness and insomnia: Association with deviated nasal septum and nocturnal breathing disorders. *Arch Otolaryngol* 1982; 108:373–377.
51. Leech HL: A clinical analysis of oro-facial morphology and behavior of 500 patients attending an upper respiratory research clinic. *Dent Pract Dent Rec* 1959; 9:88–95.
52. Leiberman A, Ohki M, Forte V, et al: Nose/mouth distribution of respiratory airflow in "mouth breathing" in children. *Acta Otolaryngol (Stockh)* 1990; 109:454–460.

53. Leiberman A, Ohki M, Cole P: The open mouth and oro-nasal breathing. *Am J Rhinol* 1991; 5(1):1–5.
54. Lugaresi E, Cirignotta F, Gerardi R, et al: Snoring and sleep apnea: Natural history of heavy snorers disease, in Guilleminault C, Partinen M (eds): *Obstructive Sleep Apnea Syndrome: Clinical Research and Treatment.* New York, Raven Press, 1990.
55. Lustro G, Stanescu D, Dooms G, et al: Hypopharyngeal and neck cross-sectional changes monitored by inductive plethysmography. *J Appl Physiol* 1990; 68(6):2649–2655.
56. Mathew OP, Abu-Osba YK, Thach BT: Response of upper airway maintaining muscles to upper airway pressure changes. *Fed Proc* 1980; 39:1074.
57. Mauer KW, Staats BA, Olsen KD: Upper airway obstruction and disordered nocturnal breathing in children. *Mayo Clin Proc* 1983; 58:349–353.
58. McBride B, Whitelaw WA: A physiological stimulus to upper airway receptors in humans. *J Appl Physiol* 1981; 51(5):1189–1197.
59. McNicholas WT, Tarlo S, Cole P, et al: Obstructive apnea during sleep in patients with seasonal allergic rhinitis. *Am Rev Respir Dis* 1982; 126:625–628.
60. McNicholas WT, Coffey M, McDonnell T, et al: Upper airway obstruction during sleep in normal subjects after selective topical oropharyngeal anesthesia. *Am Rev Respir Dis* 1987; 135:1316–1319.
61. Meredith GM: Airway and dentofacial development, in Settipane GA (ed): *Rhinitis.* Providence, RI, OceanSide Publications Inc., 1991.
62. Metes A, Ohki M, Cole P, et al: Snoring, apnea and nasal resistance in men and women. *J Otolaryngol* 1991; 20(1):57–61.
63. Metes A, Hoffstein V, Mateika S, et al: Site of airway obstruction in patients with obstructive sleep apnea before and after uveopalatopharyngoplasty. *Laryngoscope* 1991; 101(10):1102–1108.
64. Metes A, Cole P, Hoffstein V: Nasal resistance and snoring. *Laryngoscope* 1991 (in press).
65. Miljeteig H, Hoffstein V, Cole P: The effects of unilateral and bilateral nasal obstruction on snoring and sleep apnea. *Laryngoscope* (submitted for publication).
66. Miller JM, Martin RJ, Carlo WA, et al: Oral breathing in response to nasal trauma in term infants. *J Pediatr* 1987; 3(6):899–901.
67. Miller MJ, Martin RJ, Carlo WA, et al: Oral ventilation occurs in term neonates during spontaneous breathing or nasal obstruction. *Am Rev Respir Dis* 1984; 129(4):A207.
68. Niinimaa V: Cole P, Mintz S, et al: The switching point from nasal to oroasal breathing. *Respir Physiol* 1980; 42:61–71.
69. Niinimaa V: Oronasal airway choice during running. *Respir Physiol* 1983; 53:129–133.
70. Niinimaa V, Cole P, Mintz S, et al: Oronasal distribution of respiratory airflow. *Resp Physiol* 1981; 43:69–75.
71. Norton PG, Dunn EV, Haight JSJ: Snoring in adults: some epidemiological aspects. *Can Med Assoc J* 1983; 128:674–675.
72. Norton PG, Dunn EV: Snoring as a risk factor for disease: an epidemiological survey. *Br Med J* 1985; 291:630–632.

73. O'Ryan FS, Gallagher DM, LaBanc JP, et al: The relation between naso-respiratory function and dentofacial morphology: A review. *Am J Orthod* 1982; 82(5):403–410.
74. Olsen KD, Kern EB: Snoring. *Mayo Clin Proc* 1990; 65(8):1095–1105.
75. Olsen KD, Kern EB, Westbrook PR: Sleep and breathing disturbance secondary to nasal obstruction. *Otolaryngol Head Neck Surg* 1981; 89:804–810.
76. Partinen M, Guilleminault C: Evolution of obstructive sleep apnea syndrome, in Guilleminault C, Partinen M (eds): *Obstructive Sleep Apnea Syndrome: Clinical Research and Treatment.* New York, Raven Press, 1990.
77. Peter JH: Sleep apnea and cardiovascular diseases, in Guilleminault C, Partinen M (eds): *Obstructive Sleep Apnea Syndrome: Clinical Research and Treatment.* New York, Raven Press, 1990.
78. Proctor DF: The naso-oro-pharyngo-laryngeal airway. *Eur J Respir Dis* 1983; 64:89–96.
79. Powell NB, Riley RW, Guilleminault C: Maxillo-facial surgery for obstructive sleep apnea in 1990, in Guilleminault C, Partinen M (eds): *Obstructive Sleep Apnea Syndrome: Clinical Research and Treatment.* New York, Raven Press, 1990.
80. Remmers JE: Obstructive sleep apnea. *Am Rev Respir Dis* 1984; 130:153–155.
81. Richerson HB, Seebohm PM: Nasal airway response to exercise. *J Allergy* 1968:269–284.
82. Rodenstein DO, Stanescu DC: The soft palate and breathing. *Am Rev Respir Dis* 1986; 134:311–325.
83. Rodenstein DO, Stanescu DC: Absence of nasal airflow during pursed lips breathing. *Am Rev Respir Dis* 1983; 128:716–718.
84. Rodenstein DO, Kahn A, Blum D, et al: Nasal occlusion during sleep in normal and near-miss for sudden death syndrome infants. *Bull Eur Physiopathol Respir* 1987; 23:223–226.
85. Rodenstein DO, Perlmutter N, Stanescu DC: Infants are not obligatory nasal breathers. *Am Rev Respir Dis* 1985; 131:343–347.
86. Rubin AH, Phillipson EA, Lavie P: The effect of airway anesthesia on breathing in sleep. *Chest* 1983; 84(3):337–341.
87. Schmidt-Nielsen K, Bretz WL, Taylor RC: Panting in dogs. *Science* 1970; 169:1102–1104.
88. Schwartz AR, Smith PL, Wise RA, et al: Induction of upper airway occlusion in sleeping individuals with subatmospheric nasal pressure. *J Appl Physiol* 1988; 64(2):535–542.
89. Simmons FB, Hill MW: Hypersomnia caused by upper airway obstructions: A new syndrome in otolaryngology. *Ann Otol Rhinol Laryngol* 1974; 83(5):670–674.
90. Stauffer JL, Zwillich CW, Cadieux RJ, et al: Pharyngeal size and resistance in obstructive apnea. *Am Rev Respir Dis* 1987; 136:623–627.
91. Stauffer JL, Buick MK, Bixler ED, et al: Morphology of the uvula in obstructive sleep apnea. *Am Rev Respir Dis* 1989; 140(3):724–728.
92. Stocksted P, Gutierrez C: The nasal passage following rhinoplastic surgery. *J Laryngol Otol* 1983; 97:49–54.

93. Sullivan CE, Grunstein RR, Marrone O, et al: Sleep apnea-pathophysiology: Upper airway and control of breathing, in Guilleminault C, Partinen M (eds): *Obstructive Sleep Apnea Syndrome: Clinical Research and Treatment.* New York, Raven Press, 1990.
94. Sullivan CE, Issa FG, Berthon-Jones M, Eves L: Reversal of sleep apnea by continuous positive airway pressure applied through the nose. *Lancet* 1981; 1:862–865.
95. Suratt PM, McTier RF, Wilhoit SC: Collapsibility of the nasopharyngeal airway in obstructive sleep apnea. *Am Rev Respir Dis* 1985; 132:967–971.
96. Suratt PM, Dee P, Atkinson RL, et al: Fluoroscopic and computed tomographic features of the pharyngeal airway in obstructive sleep apnea. *Am Rev Respir Dis* 1983; 127(4):487–492.
97. Suratt PM, Turner BL, Wilhoit SC: Effect of intranasal obstruction on breathing during sleep. *Chest* 1986; 90:324–329.
98. Swift PGF, Emery GL: Clinical observations on response to nasal occlusion in infancy. *Arch Dis Child* 1973; 48:947–951.
99. Takagi Y, Proctor DF, Salman S, et al: Effects of cold air and carbon dioxide on nasal airflow resistance. *Ann Otolaryngol* 1969; 78:40–48.
100. Taasan V, Wynne JW, Cassisi N, et al: The effect of nasal packing on sleep, disordered breathing, and nocturnal oxygen desaturation. *Laryngoscope* 1981; 91:1163–1172.
101. Togawa K, Konno A, Miyazaka S, et al: Obstructive sleep dyspnea. Diagnosis and treatment. *Acta Otolaryngol (Stockh)* 1988; Suppl 458:167–173.
102. Ung N, Koenig J, Shapiro PA, et al: A quantitative assessment of respiratory patterns and their effects on dentofacial development. *Am J Orthod Dentofacial Orthop* 1990; 98:523–532.
103. Uddstromer M: Nasal respiration. *Acta Otolaryngol Suppl (Stockh)* 1940; 42:3–146.
104. Vig PS: Respiratory airway and orthodontics: A review of current concepts and research, in Johnston LE (ed): *Vistas in Orthodontics.* Philadelphia, Lea & Febiger, 1985.
105. Warren DW, Hairfield WM, Dalston ET: Effect of age on nasal cross-sectional area and respiratory mode in children. *Laryngoscope* 1990; 100:89–93.
106. Warren DW, Hinton VA, Hairfield WM: Measurement of nasal and oral respiration using inductive plethysmography. *Am J Orthod* 1986:480–484.
107. Watson H: The technology of inductive respiratory plethysmography. Presented at the 3rd International Symposium of Ambulatory Monitoring 1979; Clinical Research Centre, Harrow, London, England.
108. Wetmore SJ, Scrima L, Snyderman NL, et al: Post-operative evaluation of sleep apnea after uveopalatopharyngoplasty. *Laryngoscope* 1986; 96:738–741.
109. White DP, Cadieux RJ, Lombard RM, et al: The effects of nasal anesthesia on breathing during sleep. *Am Rev Respir Dis* 1985; 132:972–975.
110. Widdicombe JG, Sant' Ambrogio G, Mathew OP: Nerve receptors of the upper airway, in Mathew OP, Sant' Ambrogio G (eds): *Respiratory Function of the Upper Airway.* New York, Marcel Dekker, 1988.

111. Wilhoit SC, Suratt PM: Effect of nasal obstruction on upper airway muscle activation in normal subjects. *Chest* 1987; 92(6):1053–1055.
112. Wittig RM, Romaker A, Zorick FJ, et al: Night-to-night consistency of apneas during sleep. *Am Rev Respir Dis* 1984; 129:244–248.
113. Woodside DG, Linder-Aronson S: The channelization of upper and lower anterior face heights compared to population standards in males between 6 and 20 years. *Eur J Orthod* 1979; 1:25–40.
114. Woodside DG, Linder-Aronson S: Progressive increase in lower anterior face height and the use of the posterior occlusal bite block in its management, in Graber LW (ed): *Orthodontics, State of the Art, Essence of the Science.* St Louis, Mosby–Year Book, 1986.
115. Wright S, Haight JSJ, Zamel N, et al: Changes in pharyngeal properties after uveopalatopharyngoplasty. *Laryngoscope* 1989; 99(1):62–65.
116. Zwillich CW, Pickett C, Hanson FN, et al: Disturbed sleep and prolonged apnea during nasal obstruction in normal men. *Am Rev Respir Dis* 1981; 124:158–160.

SUGGESTED READING

1. Fairbanks DNF, Fujita S, Ikematsu T, et al (eds): *Snoring and Obstructive Sleep Apnea.* New York, Raven Press, 1987.
2. Guilleminault C, Partinen M (eds): *Obstructive Sleep Apnea Syndrome: Clinical Research and Treatment.* New York, Raven Press, 1990.
3. Mathew OP, Sant' Ambrogio G (eds): *Respiratory Function of the Upper Airway.* New York, Marcel Dekker, 1988.
4. Proctor DF, Andersen I (eds): *The Nose: Upper Airway Physiology and the Atmospheric Environment.* Amsterdam, Elsevier Biomedical Press, 1982.

CHAPTER 3

Cleansing and Conditioning

UPPER RESPIRATORY AIRFLOW

Respiratory Role of Airway Resistors

The physiologic and pathologic behavior of the resistors situated in the nasal and oral vestibules in regard to regulation of airflow, linear velocity, and distribution of nasal and oral respiratory air has been outlined in Chapters 1 and 2. The essential respiratory role of conditioning and cleansing respiratory air is dependent on airflow characteristics that are induced by these resistors and is the subject of this chapter.

As described in Chapter 1, measurements of pressure and flow of respiratory air at different sites within healthy nasal cavities have demonstrated that resistance is concentrated in the region of high-velocity flow in the anterior nose (see Figs 1–3 through 1–6). The magnitude of this nasal resistance is altered substantially by physiologic and pathologic responses of erectile mucosa to, for example, exercise or irritants, and by pharmacological responses to vasoactive substances such as topical histamine or an α-agonist. Yet, in the absence of gross structural or mucosal abnormality, the anterior location of resistance remains unchanged, and swelling of mucosa within the nasal cavum has little effect on airflow resistance of the nasal cavity by contrast with its effect in the valve region (see Figs 1–13 to 1–15).

Studies of models made from casts of fresh cadaver nasal cavities have shown linear velocity of inspiratory air during quiet breathing to approach 18 m/sec in the narrow nasal valve region[81] (see Fig 1–6). This is gale force on the Beaufort scale, and it increases to hurricane force in a sniff.[35] The airstream decelerates to 2 to 3 m/sec as it leaves the valve and enters the cavum, which, although it is a narrow slit of only 2 to 3 mm in width, has a cross-sectional area three to four times that of the valve. These dimensions and linear flow velocities may be altered by differing physiologic and pathologic nasal conditions, but the important consequences that result from orifice flow through the nasal valve and deceleration of the airstream in the cavum prevail in all but grossly abnormal circumstances (see below).

Portal Sites of Airway Resistors

The fact that the principal resistor of the breathing passages is located at the nasal respiratory portal and a resistor of similar magnitude is located at the oral portal during spontaneous mouth breathing (see Chapter 2, "Mouth Breathing") suggests that a similar function could be attributed to each. These physiologic airflow regulators impede, rather than facilitate, flow of respiratory air, but convincing evidence supports the view that their function is important and that the toll they exact in adding to the work of breathing serves a useful purpose. Among the many speculations in this vein is the proposal that breathing against upper-airway resistances generates intrathoracic pressures of physiologic importance. Resistance brakes the elastic recoil of the passive expiratory phase of breathing in resting subjects, and the resulting extended duration of expiration is thought to aid efficiency of gaseous exchange.[8, 27, 55] It is suggested also that positive airway pressures help maintain small-airway patency and oppose alveolar surface acting forces[85] as, in a more exaggerated manner, grunting, groaning, and pursed-lip breathing benefit patients with chronic obstructive pulmonary disease.[77, 83] Furthermore, it has been supposed that alternating intrathoracic respiratory pressures act as an accessory heart, which may aid blood circulation during exercise.

In addition to the physiologic significance of intrathoracic pressures generated by breathing against upper-airway resistance, there is convincing evidence that the upper-airway resistors play an essential role in conditioning and cleansing inspiratory air by ensuring that its flow characteristics are nonlaminar (as described below). Energy is required to induce and maintain inertial disturbances in the airstream, and this portion of the work of breathing is not wasted; it is indispensable for adequate modification of air in the upper airways.

FLOW CHARACTERISTICS

Disruption of Laminar Flow

As the act of inspiration draws ambient air through the nasal or oral portals into the respiratory passages, convergence of the entering airstreams promotes laminar flow.[80] If this orderly, streamlined pattern were maintained, the result would be an absence of mixing and an insulation of the respiratory mainstream of air from the mucosa by a marginal lamina—and that would restrict exchanges of heat, water, and contaminants between air and mucosa in the nose and other large respiratory passages. The real course of events in the upper airways, however, is very different from this scenario. In this portion of the respiratory tract, where thermal and water-vapor pressure gradients between mucosa and inspiratory air are high, there are several features of inspiratory airflow and of the upper-airway passages themselves that make it improbable that laminar-flow regimens of inspiratory air could prevail beyond the nasal valve. Only briefly, near the beginning and end of each inspiratory and expiratory breath, is the linear velocity of the airstream conducive to laminar flow (Reynolds). In addition, respiratory flow is repeatedly accelerating, then decelerating, and then reversing again. It changes direction through 180° between the anterior nares and the pharynx and flows through a lumen of varying shape and cross-sectional dimension, most marked by narrowing at the nasal valve. All these features impose disturbances on the flow pattern of the inspiratory airstream.

As inspiratory air leaves the narrow nasal valve and enters the much larger nasal cavum, its linear velocity is substantially reduced (see Fig 1–6). Kinetic energy of the airstream, which is exponentially related to its velocity ($E = kv^2$), is released on deceleration and dissipated in the generation of inertial flow disturbances. Thus, the orderly laminar pattern is destabilized and its marginal lamina is disrupted. The non-laminar regime may be transitional or, beyond a critical velocity, turbulent (see below). The nasally induced flow disturbances are reinforced by pharyngeal and glottic narrowings[23] and entrained to the bronchi.[9] They bring about mucosal contact and mixing essential for effective modification of air in its brief passage through the large-diameter upper airways.[43] Oral and nasal vestibules function in a similar manner; and, indeed, the oral cavity has the capacity for conditioning and cleansing inspiratory air as effectively as the nasal cavities in resting and moderately exercising subjects.[21, 39, 40–42]

Turbulence and Nasal Resistance

Nasal resistance to air breathing is lowered by lesser-density helium mixtures,[15] and the sigmoid shape of the respiratory transnasal pressure-flow curve approaches a straight line. Experiments with other chemically inert gas mixtures (e.g, sulfur hexafluoride) have shown that turbulence and nasal resistance to flow are positively correlated with gas density and with its linear velocity.[32]

Not only is laminar flow disrupted by the nasal valve orifice, but frictional forces in the air passages induce disturbance and maintain non-laminar flow. If the linear velocity of a fluid in a conduit increases from zero, the equation $P = \text{k}V^e$ (exponent $e = 1$) describes the initial pressure-flow ratio. As velocity increases, frictional forces increase also and generate inertial flow disturbances. Initial laminar-flow characteristics are replaced, and the exponent e becomes > 1. The flow regime of the phase in which the disturbances are introduced is termed *transitional,* and the disturbances increase, together with linear velocity, until, at a critical velocity, full turbulence is achieved (Reynolds). Turbulence can be described mathematically in terms of pressure and flow, with the exponent e approaching 2,[66] but *transitional* characterizes the prevalent respiratory-flow regime in the upper airways of subjects at rest.[45] Several investigators have advocated use of an exponent <2 to describe lesser degrees of flow disturbance and to fit transnasal pressure-flow data. Curve-fitting and estimations of the slope of logarithmic plots of transnasal pressure against flow have suggested exponent e to lie in the range of 1.6 to 1.8.

Laser anemometry shows the nasal valve to direct the inspiratory airstream with its greatest velocity along the septum, and velocity fields and profiles demonstrate turbulent flow under circumstances in which turbulence could not be demonstrated by application of Reynold's calculation.[28] It is of surgical interest also that, as mentioned in Chapter 1, "Nasal Valve," obstruction of the apical portion of the nasal valve has little effect on airflow resistance, respiratory air flows mainly through its basal portion (Cole, Haight, and Chaban, unpublished, 1990).

Increase in velocity of airflow, like the ventilation of exercise, reduces duration of exposure of respiratory air to mucosa in each conducting segment of the airways, but as linear velocities are increased, greater airflow disturbances that enhance mucosal contact and mixing are induced also (Reynolds). They compensate to some degree for the reduction in transit time. Furthermore, greater energy of these reinforced disturbances enables them to be entrained more deeply into the air passages than those induced by spontaneous breathing at rest. Greater penetration of the disturbances to more peripheral airways[9] augments the mucosal area exposed to flow conditions that are conducive to convective transfer of heat, water, and contaminants.

Exercise increases flow of respiratory air, and, by decongestion of erectile tissues (see Chapter 1, "Erectile Mucosa"), cross section of the nasal valve and cavum are increased also. Thus, although impedence to airflow is diminished, orifice flow and increased linear velocity sustain disruption of the laminar pattern of the airstream, and it seems that the oral airway and the labial resistor behave in a similar manner (see Chapter 2, "Mouth Breathing").

Nasal Airflow Recording

Pneumotachograms, which record respiratory airflow over time (Fig 3–1), demonstrate a square inspiratory waveform in subjects breathing nasally at rest. In other words, maximum inspiratory flow is maintained through most of the inspiratory phase. This rate of flow through the nasal valve ensures that non-laminar flow will prevail in the upper airways through most of the inspiratory phase of the breathing cycle. By contrast, the expiratory

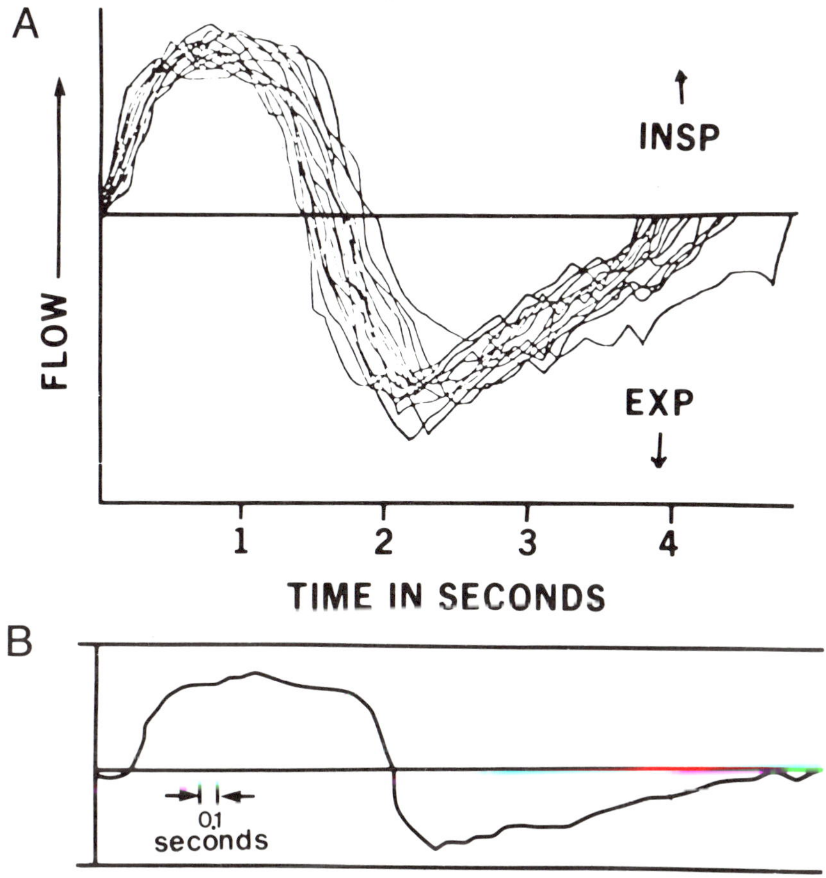

FIG 3–1.

A, pneumotachograms of several breaths of a subject at rest. **B,** representation of a single breath. Note squarish form of inspiratory tracing and linear slope from peak to zero of expiration. (From Proctor DF, Hardy JB: Studies of respiratory airflow. *Bull Johns Hopkins Hosp* 1949; 85:253. Used by permission.)

waveform of subjects breathing at rest falls in linear fashion from its peak to zero as passive elastic recoil of the tissues obeys Hooke's Law (refer again to Fig 3–1). Expiration against applied airway resistance and the increased ventilation of exercise requires muscular effort to augment respiratory forces, and the muscular effort imposes a square configuration on the expiratory wave also[65] (Fig 3–2). Thus, the proportion of the breathing cycle occupied by plateaus of inspiratory and expiratory phases increases with ventilatory effort. The squaring of the pneumotachogram waveform repre-

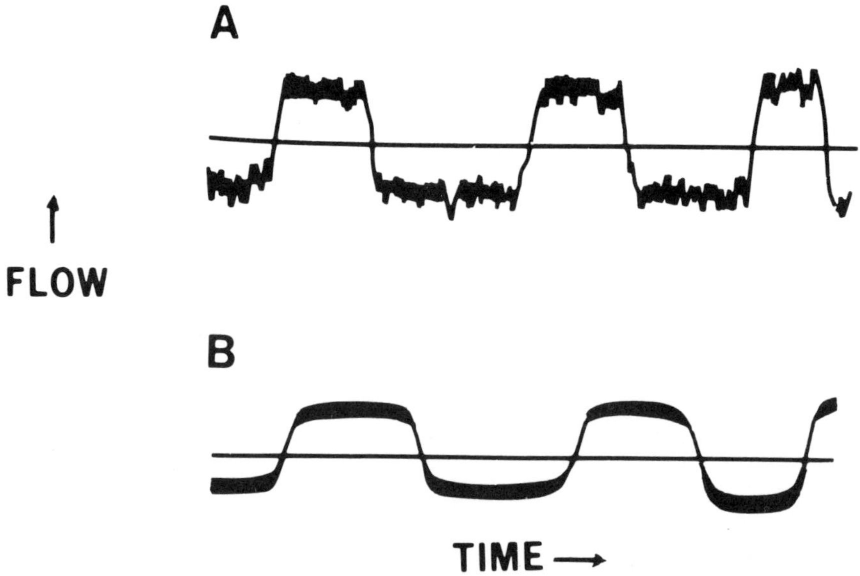

FIG 3–2.
A, pneumotachogram of a subject during exercise. **B,** the same subject is breathing against applied resistance. Note square configuration of both representations. (From Proctor DF, Hardy JB: Studies of respiratory airflow. *Bull Johns Hopkins Hosp* 1949; 85:253. Used by permission.)

sents physiologic optimization of the efficiency of both the muscular work of breathing and of air modification.[47]

The pneumotachogram that represents respiratory airflow has complex determinants, and its configuration varies among subjects and according to respiratory health, but it is identical at all points in an individual subject's extrapulmonary airway beyond the carina during either exclusive nasal or oral breathing. By contrast, linear-flow velocities and differential pressure profiles are not identical; they are characteristic of each airway segment and are amplified at the airway portals and at other narrowed sites. The exponential relationship between differential pressures and linear-flow velocities contributes to the sigmoid shape of the pressure-flow curve (Fig 3–3).

Several early reports have indicated a preferential pulmonary distribution of inspiratory airflow (e.g., right nostril, right lung),[68] but radioactive krypton gas inhaled through a single nostril has been found uniformly mixed in the tracheal airstream.[51] Similar results were obtained with xenon-133 gas studies that showed neither preferential streaming nor the reflex bronchoconstriction that had been reported to accompany nasal obstruction.[77] In addition, lung function has been found not to reflect the alternating airflow resistances of the nasal cycle.[75]

Nasal Patency

Studies of nasal patency are commonly undertaken by means of an x-y plot of transnasal pressures against respiratory airflow during exclusive nasal breathing (see Chapter 4, "Objective Measurement"). The plot produces a sigmoid tracing (see Fig 3–3) that has received numerous mathematical descriptions. Rohrer's equation, $P = k_1\dot{V} + k_2\dot{V}^2$ has endured since 1915, and several different transforms and polynomial descriptions have been advocated as well. Although Rohrer's equation is widely used, it has many critics.[72] It is said to include a dimensional error, and correction by a factor of one-tenth reduces the importance of its first term.[86] Authorities disagree as to the significance of the constants k_1 *and* k_2.[54, 82] Also, gas density and viscosity effects do not fit the equation,[45] and it has been stated that curve-fitting does not justify its use.[61] Some have argued that a polynomial

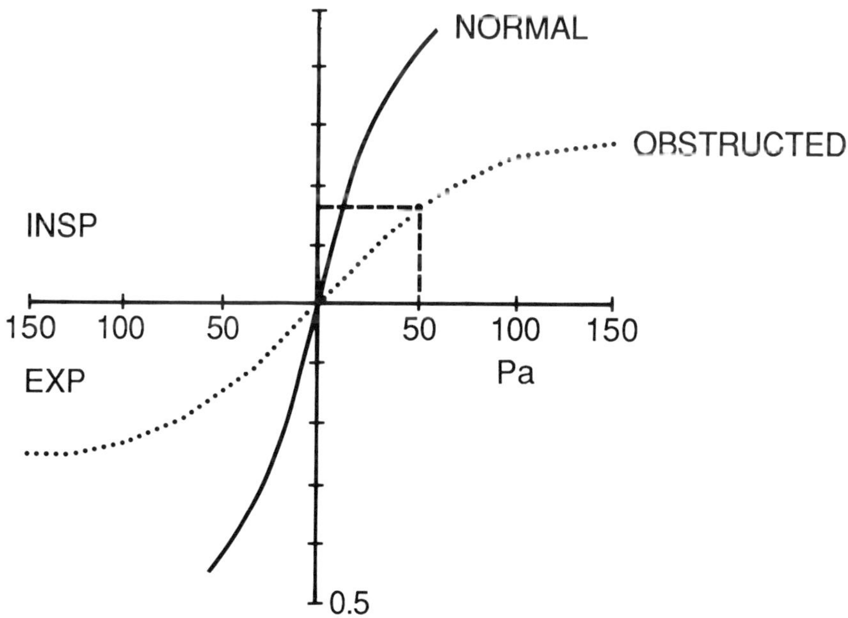

FIG 3–3.

Transnasal pressure-flow curves of a normal and a nasally obstructed subject breathing at rest. Note sigmoid shape of the curves and their rotation toward the pressure axis as resistance is increased.

requires >3 terms to describe the respiratory transnasal pressure-flow curve, while others deem application of Bernoulli's equation to flow through the nasal-valve orifice adequate.[62]

Traditionally, the sigmoid shape of the pressure-flow curve is interpreted as representing laminar flow in its straighter portion (in the vicinity of the origin) and turbulent flow in its more curvilinear portion (distant from the origin). On the other hand, close curve-fitting results also from calculating resistances by application of Bernoulli's equation to airflow through models of the nasal-valve orifice.[62] It is argued that application of Reynold's equation to nasal airflow is inappropriate, and the situation as described by that of Bernoulli is consistent with results of several investigations that localize the major portion of nasal airflow resistance to the valve.

Although inspiratory and expiratory phases of the pressure-flow curve are assumed to be symmetrical by some investigators, observation shows this not to be the case in all subjects breathing spontaneously at rest[72, 73] (Fig 3–4,A). Rather, the expiratory limb is sometimes attenuated. Symmetry that is approached as ventilation (Fig 3–4,B) or resistance is increased is demonstrated clearly by the pneumotachograph studies shown in Figures 3–1 and 3–2. It is probable that in many cases of pressure-flow recording by means of a mask or nasal nozzle, ventilation is elevated for a variety of reasons despite the subject being seated and at rest,[6, 36] and increased tidal flow causes the tracing to assume a more symmetrical appearance (see Fig 3–4,B again).

Pressure-flow recordings do not include a time scale. Consequently, duration of flow rates, accelerations, and decelerations are not displayed by this form of recording. But direct observation of the moving spot on an oscilloscope or monitor screen shows it to linger near the extremities of the pressure-flow tracing (digital recordings show an accumulation of data points at the extremities), thereby reflecting duration of the plateaus of the breathing pattern. Some investigations suggest that these features may have a bearing on sensation of nasal patency[59] and are better displayed by the flow-time and pressure-time methods of charting that were customary in earlier rhinomanometric techniques.[22]

Clinical comment: Despite the complex features of upper respiratory airflow and many uncertainties, indices of nasal patency derived empirically from transnasal pressure and flow values are widely used as practical clinical and experimental measures and are discussed in Chapter 4 under "Indices of Nasal Patency" and "Clinical Rhinomanometry."

A

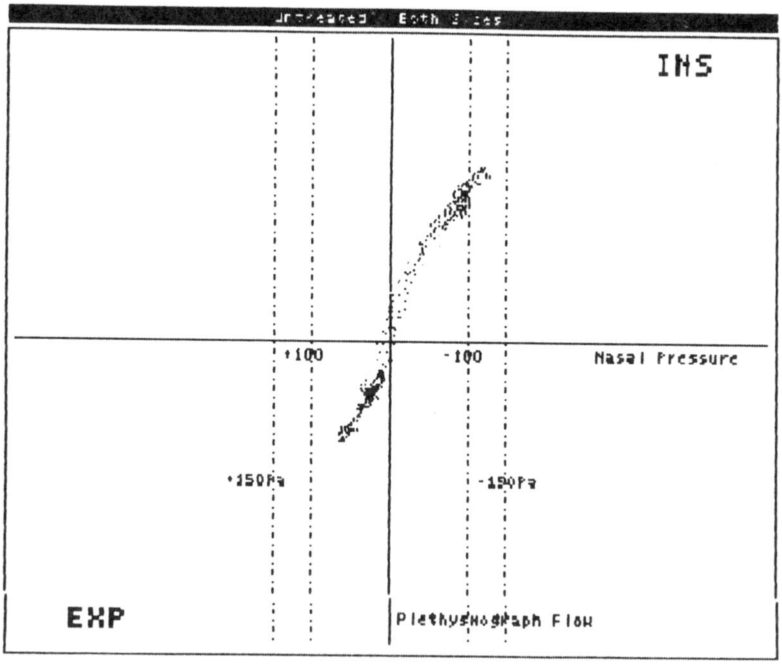

B

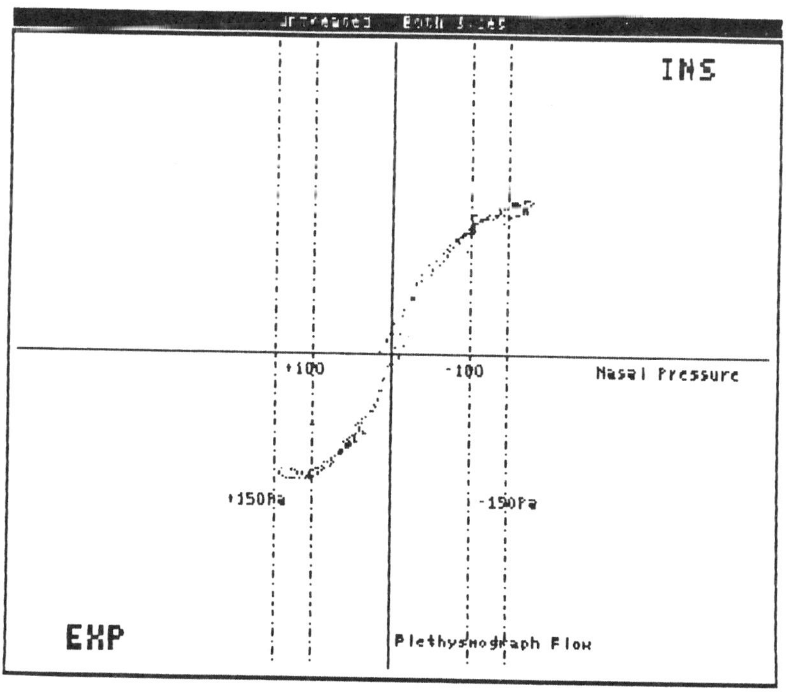

FIG 3–4.

Transnasal pressure-flow curves of a subject breathing spontaneously at rest **(A)** (note asymmetry) and with voluntary increase in tidal ventilation **(B)** (note increase in symmetry).

Oral Breathing

Descriptions of the airflow characteristics of nasal breathing apply also to oral breathing. The spontaneously positioned resistive labial aperture induces inertial disturbance in the inspiratory airstream, thus ensuring disruption of laminar flow. As discussed a little later in this chapter, the temperature, humidity, and other modifications achieved by inspiratory air at laryngeal level are similar during either nasal or oral breathing.[16, 39, 41]

Upper and Lower Airways Compared

There are striking differences between respiratory airflow characteristics in the extrapulmonary airways and those in the air passages within the lungs. Distances between midstream and mucosa in the extrapulmonary airways is as great as several millimeters in some segments, and mass movement of air is parallel with the walls of the segment. In order to maximize exchanges of heat, water, and pollutants, the airflow velocities perpendicular to the mainstream must be maximized also. Disruption of laminar flow as described above is essential to this end, and it enables substantial conditioning of inspiratory air to be attained before the air reaches the small intrapulmonary passages.[42, 43]

These small pulmonary air passages of 2 mm diameter and less are generated to many thousands by 25 or more subdivisions. In their lumen, linear velocity of respiratory airflow is reduced by a factor of 1,000,[45] and the mainstream is close to mucosa that has a surface area 1,000 times greater than 150 cm^2 of the nose. Here diffusion[26] plays a greater part in thermal and aqueous exchanges than the convective transfer characteristics that predominate in the larger extrapulmonary air passages.

In the lower airways, languid flow is linearly related to small differential pressures, and its characteristics are laminar. In the upper airways, turbulence, velocity, resistance, and energy of airflow are high, and the relationship between flow and pressure is exponential. Indeed, the greater portion of energy expended on respiratory airflow is dissipated in the extrapulmonary airways.

AIR CONDITIONING

Ambient to Alveolar Air Conditioning

The upper airways serve and protect the peripheral pulmonary airways over a wide range of ambient conditions that would be hostile to the delicate epithelium of terminal air passages and alveoli and would impair their function. As an example of an effect of environmental exposure, specialized ciliated columnar cells of respiratory epithelium in the anterior nose are replaced by transition to simpler "wear and tear" cuboidal and squamous forms.[5]

The upper airways cleanse, warm, and moisten inspiratory air and, together with the more central lower conducting airways, where conditioning deficiencies are reduced further, they help maintain an alveolar environment in which the temperature, humidity, and freedom from harmful substances are optimal for exchanges of oxygen and carbon dioxide.

Nasal Air Conditioning

Inspiratory air conditioning that takes place in the nasal cavities is frequently presented as a remarkable accomplishment of nasal function. However, the phenomenon of effective air conditioning can be viewed from another perspective: the rapid uptake of heat and water by the airstream can be regarded as a manifestation of the thermal properties and flow characteristics of the air itself. Indeed, under suitable circumstances, transfer of heat and water takes place with great readiness between cool, dry air and warm, moist surfaces, and vice versa.

Conditioning can be achieved as effectively as in the nasal cavities by an entirely inanimate apparatus consisting of a plain glass tube containing moist paper pellets. A simple experiment has been performed in which a subject, with a nose clip occluding the nasal airways, breathes via the mouth through such a tube.[18] Measurements of inspiratory air temperature and humidity at the proximal end of the tube, before the air reaches the mouth, demonstrate that it is conditioned as effectively by this uncomplicated apparatus as inspiratory air reaching the nasopharynx is conditioned by passage through the nasal cavities (Table 3–1). Apparently, the moist paper pellets in the lumen of the tube impede airflow and induce flow disturbances of respiratory air. These disturbances ensure mixing and contact with exposed surfaces, and expiratory air gives up specific heat, moisture, and latent heat of vaporization to be picked up by the inspiratory airstream. More sophisticated heat-and-moisture exchangers that employ similar principles have been manufactured for clinical use.[63]

TABLE 3–1.
Inspiratory Air Temperature at Airway Sites (°C)

	Portal	Pharynx	Subglottis	Trachea	Carina
Nasal breathing	20	31	33	35	36
Tracheostomal breathing	20	–	–	30	32

Countercurrent Heat and Water Exchanges

There are many examples of heat and water exchange by this countercurrent principle in both live (discussed later) and artificial airways. It is probable that under the extreme conditions of temperature, humidity, and ventilation experienced by high-altitude climbers,[37] breathing apparatus is successful not only because it oxygenates the blood, but also retains large amounts of heat and water within the breathing system which would otherwise be lost by the climber.

Endotracheal intubation and attached anesthetic tubing can adequately replace the nose as a conditioner of inspiratory air,[24] but restriction of this important avenue of heat loss in expiratory air can be detrimental. Anesthetic tubing that acts as a heat exchanger also restricts heat losses in expiratory air.[14, 24] Under circumstances in which other routes are restricted also, or thermoregulatory mechanisms are impaired—as might occur during lengthy periods of general anesthesia in a humid operating room with a blanketed patient—respiratory heat retention might contribute to hyperthermia and thus constitute a danger to the patient.

Circumstances That Aid Air Conditioning

As already described, air conditioning takes place very readily when appropriate circumstances prevail. Laryngectomized patients, whose permanent tracheal breathing bypasses the nose, mouth, and pharynx, cope reasonably well with their environment, and measurements have shown that air temperatures at the carina are similar to those in the pharynx of nasally breathing subjects.[33, 34] Circumstances for air conditioning are particularly favorable in the nasal cavities. These airway segments are narrowed to a slit 2 to 3 mm wide, the midstream is close to mucosa, temperature and water-vapor pressure gradients are higher than elsewhere in the respiratory passages, and flow disturbances that promote mucosal contact and mixing are induced by the nasal valve. Sources of heat required for exchanges with inspiratory air are provided by recovery from expiratory air and from blood circulating through the mucosa.

It is not surprising that in these favorable situations, inspiratory air accumulates heat and water vapor and deposits contaminants, accomplishing a substantial proportion of the conditioning as the air passes through the nose to the pharynx. Nevertheless, conditioning of inspiratory air that reaches the pharynx during nasal (or oral) breathing is still incomplete. Although saturated with water vapor, the air has not achieved alveolar temperature (Fig 3–5; also see Table 3–1). Further increases in temperature take place as inspiratory air proceeds more deeply into the air passages, along with a rapid uptake of exponentially greater quantities of water that maintain saturation (see Fig 3–5). Specific heat of air is small and, except in extremely low ambient temperatures, the major thermal demand by inspiratory air is for supply of latent heat necessary to vaporize water from the mucosal surface (540 calories/gm) in order to saturate the air with water vapor.

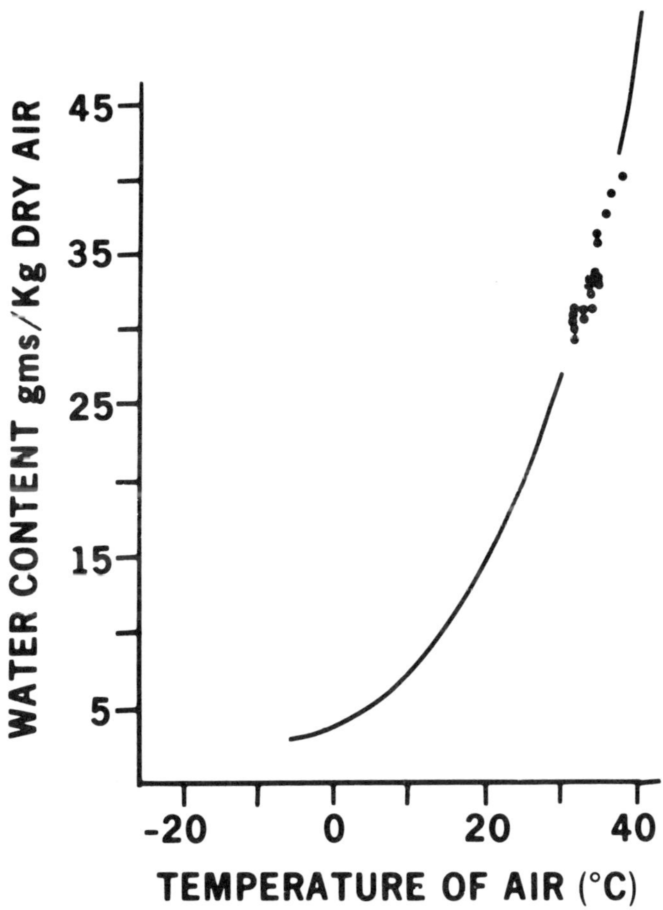

FIG 3–5.

Water required to saturate air increases exponentially with temperature. Points on the curve represent pharyngeal inspiratory air temperature and 100% saturation during nasal breathing under differing ambient conditions. Note full saturation at whatever temperature is achieved on passage of inspiratory air through the nose. (From Cole P: Further observations on conditioning of respiratory air. *J Laryngol* 1953; 67:669. Used by permission.)

Blood-borne Heat

It has been suggested that nasal mucosal blood flow adjusts, by increasing or decreasing, in order to supply rapidly altered thermal requirements of inspiratory air that result from ambient changes of temperature and humidity or of ventilation. However, efforts to demonstrate an inverse relationship between inspiratory air temperature and nasal mucosal blood flow have been unsuccessful. Moreover, it has been shown (Olsson and Bende, personal communication, 1990), and is discussed later in this chapter, that nasal mucosal blood flow, like that of the skin, varies directly with the temperature of acute local and remote thermal stimuli.

An alternative exists to the idea that nasal mucosal blood flow accommodates changes in the thermal requirements of respiratory air conditioning. The inanimate heat-and-moisture exchanger described earlier extracts sufficient heat from expiratory air to condition the inspiratory airstream effectively; and since similar airflow characteristics prevail in the respiratory airways, it could be argued that blood-borne heat from the nasal mucosa is less than essential for conditioning inspiratory air. Furthermore, in exercising subjects, whose thermal demands for maintenance of optimum alveolar temperature and humidity are high, oronasal breathing diverts much of the respiratory air through the mouth. Thus, the thermal-exchange potential of blood-borne heat of the nasal mucosa is only partially exploited; had it been essential, it is unlikely that it would be abandoned so readily.

As shown below, increasing thermal demands are met, at least in the short term, by increasing the area of respiratory-tract mucosa that is involved in air conditioning. In other words, air conditioning to any specific degree extends more deeply into the air passages as thermal demands increase. Much of the heat transferred to inspiratory air is recovered from expiratory air (see "Heat and Water Recovery" later in this chapter), and the remaining portion is blood-borne. Yet, the lively behavior of nasal mucosal blood flow that has been demonstrated in response to ambient and other factors appears less appropriately devoted to heating inspiratory air than to regulating the condition of expiratory air, and thus playing a part in heat and water economy (see "Thermoregulation" near the end of this chapter).

AIR CLEANSING

Cleansing by Nasal and Oral Air Passages

The atmosphere is a sink and a cesspool. In urban environments, in homes, and in workplaces, it is a common source of toxic substances[1] with a potential for injuring healthy air passages and worsening the function and condition of those already unhealthy.[78, 79] The airflow characteristics described in this chapter play an essential role not only in heat and moisture transfer, but also in removal of water-soluble and particulate contaminants from inspiratory air. Particulates that impinge on the mucosal surface are entrapped in mucus and transported to the pharynx by metachronal ciliary activity in the rigid portions of the airway and are swallowed. The fate of water-soluble contaminants is less certain; it seems likely that a fraction would follow the same route.

Major factors that influence removal of particulates from the airstream and their depth of penetration into the air passages include particle size, velocity, and turbulence of the airstream, and configuration of the air passages. Although atmospheric debris is deposited in the nasal vestibule, vibrissae are commonly absent or scanty and are unlikely to provide an essential filtering function. Vibrissae differ from body hairs in their lack of arrector pili muscles and they are sensitive to mechanical stimulation. Their displacement warns of invasion of a nasal cavity that is guarded by an incomplete sphincter and initiates further protection by the sneeze reflex.

Controlled chamber studies of healthy subjects exposed to inert dust (particles of 1.8 to 12.5 μm) have been performed. These experiments show that during resting nasal ventilation, 55% of small and 20% of large particles remain in the inspiratory pharyngeal airstream.[3] It is reported also that 100% of 15μm particles and only 5% of 1μm particles are deposited in the nasal cavities.[76] Beyond the nasal cavities, the airstream makes an abrupt change in direction, and the nasopharynx is a major site of deposition. Particulate penetration increases with flow velocity despite increasing disturbances in the airstream. Very small particles can remain suspended as far as the alveoli, and they have been detected in expiratory air.

Similar comments apply to inhalation of gaseous contaminants. Lesser solubilities, greater concentrations, and increased airflow velocities augment penetration, but extended duration of exposure has been found not to diminish effective removal of air pollutants in the nose.[2] Sulfur dioxide, ammonia, hydrochloric acid, and formaldehyde are water-soluble and thus are effectively removed from the airstream within the nasal cavities. Nitrogen oxides are less soluble and thus less completely removed, and carbon monoxide and hydrocarbons are not removed at all.[11] Chemical reactivity plays a part in removal of substances such as the photochemical air pollutant, ozone. Although this gas is not very soluble, 40% is removed in the nose.[64] Experimentally high concentrations have been shown to penetrate deeply and to injure peripheral pulmonary airways of animals and also to impair pulmonary function in humans.[78, 79]

The mouth also is an effective cleanser of inspiratory air, but a mouthpiece, as commonly used in experimental work, eliminates the labial resistor (see Chapter 2, "Mouth Breathing") and complicates interpretation of the spontaneous efficiency of the mouth as an air scrubber. More realistic measurements that have avoided invasion by a mouthpiece suggest the mouth can be as effective as the nose in protecting the lower airways.[21, 39, 46]

HEAT AND WATER TRANSFER

Gradient From Portal to Alveolus

The picture that is sometimes presented of conditioning and cleansing of inspiratory air nearing completion in the nasal passages is misleading. These processes commence in the nasal or oral cavities and continue to the peripheral pulmonary airways. Convolutions of the nasal mucosa expand its area, but to only 150 cm^2 in humans, and the warm, moist areas of the mouth exposed to the airstream are of similar size. These areas are miniscule by comparison with the mucosal area of the peripheral airways.

It should be noted also that although the most striking vascular structures of the turbinates are the extensive arrays of capacitance (not exchange) vessels, attempts to compare the functional importance of these vessels with radiators or with the heat-exchanger tubes of a steam generator, are unrealistic. The function of turbinate capacitance vessels is to contain rather than conduct blood, and thereby to adjust nasal lumen. Numerous arteriovenous shunts in the nasal mucosa, as in the skin,[13, 31, 50] are concerned with heat transfer that takes place by convection. Radiation is unlikely to play a significant thermal role in nasal air conditioning.

Limitations of Nasal Air Conditioning

Pharyngeal air temperature measurements show that the limits of nasal mucosal heat transfer are exceeded with every breath (Fig 3–6; see also Table 3–1). Nevertheless, although incomplete, a substantial proportion of inspiratory air conditioning takes place in the nose and the large-diameter extrapulmonary airways by exchanges between a relatively small mucosal area and a rapidly moving "turbulent" (non-laminar) airstream by convective transfer. Conditioning then approaches completion in increasingly

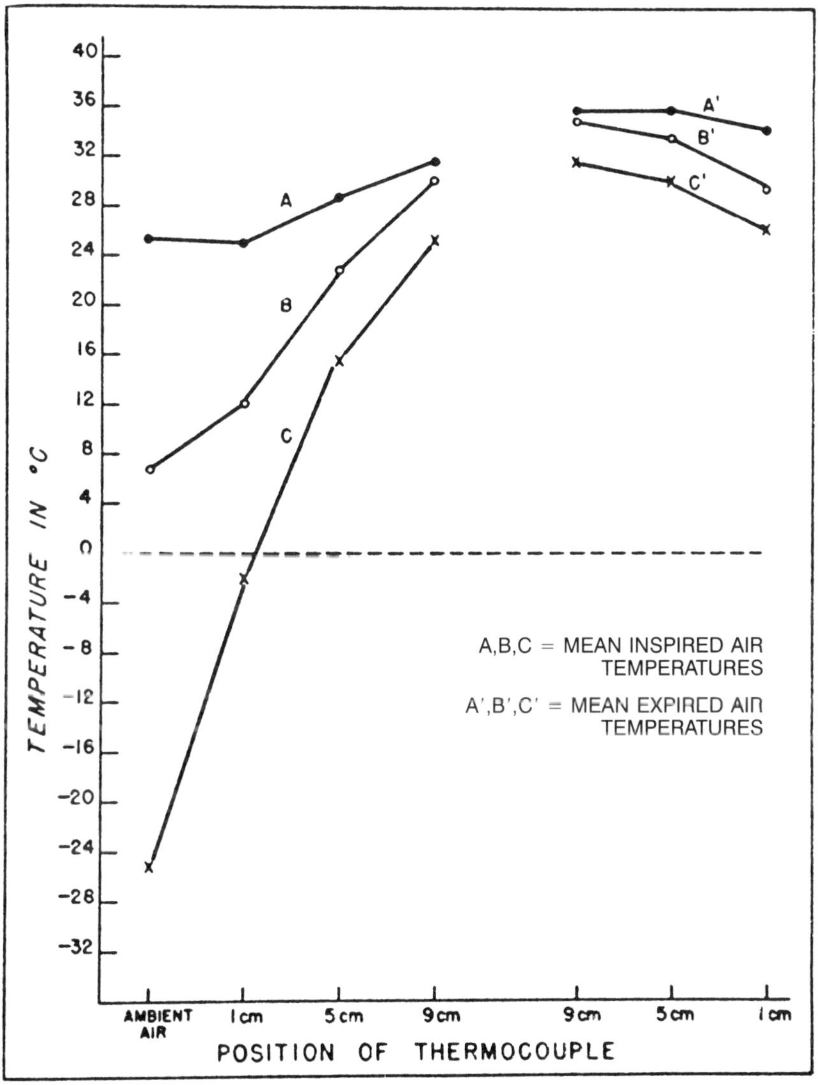

FIG 3–6.

Temperatures of inspiratory and expiratory air at nasal sites under differing ambient conditions. Note that conditioning of inspiratory air by the nasal passages is incomplete and expiratory air is below core temperature in the pharynx. Air is cooled further on passing through the nose. (From Webb P: Air temperature in the respiratory tracts of resting subjects in the cold. *J Appl Physiol* 1951; 4:378. Used by permission.)

smaller and more numerous peripheral airways where slowly moving air is intimately exposed to a very large mucosal area.

Increasing demands by ventilation of exercise or by ambient extremes are met by deeper penetration of incompletely conditioned inspiratory air, with exposure to an increased area of mucosa in order to achieve a given condition. As the conditioning processes infiltrate peripherally, substantial thermal reserves of the enormous mucosal area of the small conducting airways accommodate them and minimizes disturbance of air condition in the terminal bronchioles and alveoli. By these means, as inspiratory air proceeds peripherally, increasing resources are brought to bear on decreasing requirements of heat and water transfer, and a substantial thermal buffer of small-airway mucosa ensures that modification of inspiratory air, with its well-conditioned dead-space component, approaches completion as it nears the periphery. On reaching its termination, inspiratory air mixes with the large volume of well-conditioned residual air that provides an additional thermal buffer.

Extreme Exposures

Acute exposure to extreme conditions of inspiratory air has shown no significant effect on pulmonary blood temperature in animal studies.[29, 52, 67] Exposure of dogs to inspiratory air at extremes of temperature (−100 to +550° C) conducted through an insulated endotracheal tube has demonstrated that airway injury is confined to the large central conducting air passages, sparing those in the periphery.[56] Clinical findings reported in World War II aircrew members following exposure to extreme conditions as a consequence of aircraft damage in flight are consistent with the results of animal studies. It seems that the peripheral airways and alveoli are well protected by the processing of inspiratory air in the upper and central conducting passages, and even most severe exposures result in minimal disturbances of temperature and humidity in the terminal air passages.

By contrast, a study of chronic exposure to extreme cold in the Canadian arctic has attributed the prevalence of obstructive pulmonary disease among the Inuit people to thermal injury. The investigators note that it seems unlikely to be a result of cigarette smoking since progress of the disease is suspended during lengthy convalescent periods in a sanitarium where smoking was unrestricted, but the climate was more benign. These findings suggest the possibility that there are limits to the protection afforded by the upper airways against injury from penetration of arctic air. Russian investigators also have reported pathologic pulmonary findings in circumpolar hunters.[69]

Recordings of air and mucosal temperatures extending from the upper airways to subsegmental bronchi have been obtained in acute experiments from human volunteers exposed to extreme conditions of temperature, humidity, and ventilation,[17, 18, 19, 53] but these acute experiments may not be entirely representative of chronic situations.

Under temperate conditions, the nasal airways of healthy subjects at rest will warm inspiratory air to 31 to 32° C. As the air proceeds through the pharynx to the subglottic region, it gains heat and its temperature increases to 33 to 34° C. This process continues in the trachea, and at the carina an air temperature of 36° C is achieved. In subsegmental bronchi, the temperature is little different from that of the alveoli and the body core (see Table 3–1 and Figure 3–6).

As the system is stressed by increased ventilation, by temperature and humidity extremes, or a combination of these factors, the pharyngeal inspiratory air temperatures cited above are found more peripherally in the airways. Air temperatures as low as 28° C have been recorded in subsegmental bronchi of subjects exposed to extreme experimental conditions,[53] and under these circumstances pharyngeal and tracheal temperatures are correspondingly lower also.

Mucosal Temperatures

Alveolar and terminal bronchiolar air and mucosa maintain a temperature of 37° C, and average temperatures decrease as the airway portal is approached[24] (Fig 3–7). At the nasal portal, average mucosal and expiratory air temperatures of 31 to 32° C prevail in temperate conditions. Temperature swings within the airways between inspiratory and expiratory phases are augmented by thermal demands, and their amplitude decreases as the periphery and a temperature of 37° C are approached (see Fig 3–7). Thermal effects of cold air are not confined to the mucosal surface of the airways but are conducted to surrounding tissues, and they are reflected in esophageal temperature measurements.[30, 44]

The limitations of blood-borne heat supply to respiratory mucosa in response to thermal demands of inspiratory air are exemplified by these low air and tissue temperatures and by the sluggish rewarming of turbinate tissue on cessation of nasal breathing (see next section in this chapter and Fig 3–8). Investigation of exercise-induced asthma that has stimulated many of these experiments has revealed remarkably low temperatures of air and of mucosa deep within the air passages, but there is disagreement among pulmonary respirologists as to whether bronchospasm results from thermal effects of low temperature or from osmotic effects of evaporation of mucosal water.

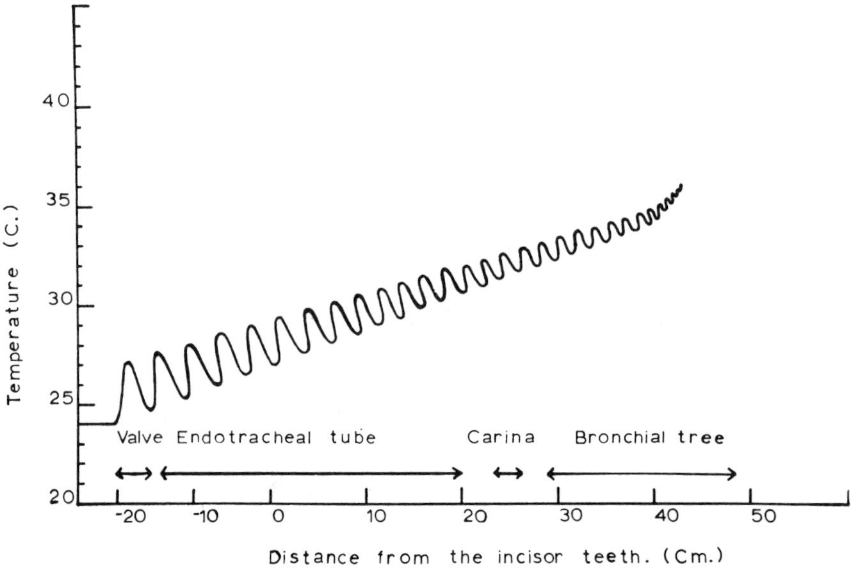

FIG 3–7.
Temperature swings in respiratory air are reduced as it approaches the periphery and 37° C. (From Dery R, Pelletier J, Jacques A, et al: Humidity in anaesthesiology. *Can Anaesth Soc J* 1967; 14:287. Used by permission.)

Water Vapor

Measurements of the water content of respiratory air have shown repeatedly that within the air passages it is saturated (see Fig 3–5). Evaporation and condensation are almost immediate accompaniments of temperature change.[12, 18, 25, 49] As mentioned above, in all but the most severely cold conditions the major portion of thermal energy required for air modification is spent in the supply of latent heat of vaporization.

Figure 3–5 shows the exponential relationship between air temperature and the quantity of water required for saturation. The saturation curve is steep in the region of body temperature, meaning that small changes in temperature of air within the respiratory passages result in large changes in its water content, and correspondingly large changes in its latent heat content. It is of clinical interest to note from this figure how small a contribution to humidification of air at body temperature (37° C) is achieved as air is bubbled through water at room temperature (<25% at 20° C).

Water has been termed "nature's thermostat." Both latent heat of vaporization and specific heat of water are far greater than in other substances, and these properties protect the peripheral airways from thermal damage (specific heat of air is very small) by providing a large caloric reservoir (or sink) for rapid moderation of extreme inspiratory air conditions. With the possible exception of chronic exposure to extremes of ventilation in polar regions, it seems unlikely that terminal airways could suffer thermal injury or desiccation.

HEAT AND WATER RECOVERY

Cooling and Condensation

Measurements of expiratory air condition demonstrate that although fully saturated with water, its temperature is lower than that of the body.[49] It was supposed at one time that body temperature was never fully achieved by respiratory air. It is now recognized that as expiratory air leaves the periphery, it comes into contact with mucosal surfaces that are cooled by inspiratory air and incompletely warmed by circulating blood. Expiratory air releases heat and water by condensation on the cooled mucosal surfaces and thus contributes to the conditioning of inspiratory air (see Fig 3–6). Mean values of mucosal surface temperatures that fluctuate with the respiratory cycle become increasingly lower than that of the body core as the airway portal is approached. They are representative of the thermal equilibrium resulting from (1) heat transferred to inspiratory air and (2) heat supplied by both circulating blood and by recovery from expiratory air.

A microthermometer inserted deep to the surface of the human turbinate submucosa shows no cyclical fluctuation with respiration from 32° C in temperate room conditions (Fig 3–8). On cessation of nasal breathing, several minutes elapse before body temperature is attained, indicating that conduction of blood-borne heat by turbinate tissue is not a very rapid process. The mucosa remains below body temperature throughout the breathing cycle, enabling the recovery process in humans to retrieve about 30% of the heat and water from expiratory air in temperate conditions.

Recovery takes place throughout the airways, but the nasal cavities play the major role during nasal breathing, and partial closure of the glottis in expiration produces orifice flow that promotes convective exchanges. Expiratory heat and water losses are greater during oral or tracheostomal breathing, as they are in pyrexial patients, and a water loss as great as 4 liters in 24 hours has been reported in a pyrexial patient breathing through a tracheal stoma.[84]

Breathing colder or drier air increases recovery. The converse is found with warmer and more humid conditions. The increase in nasal airflow

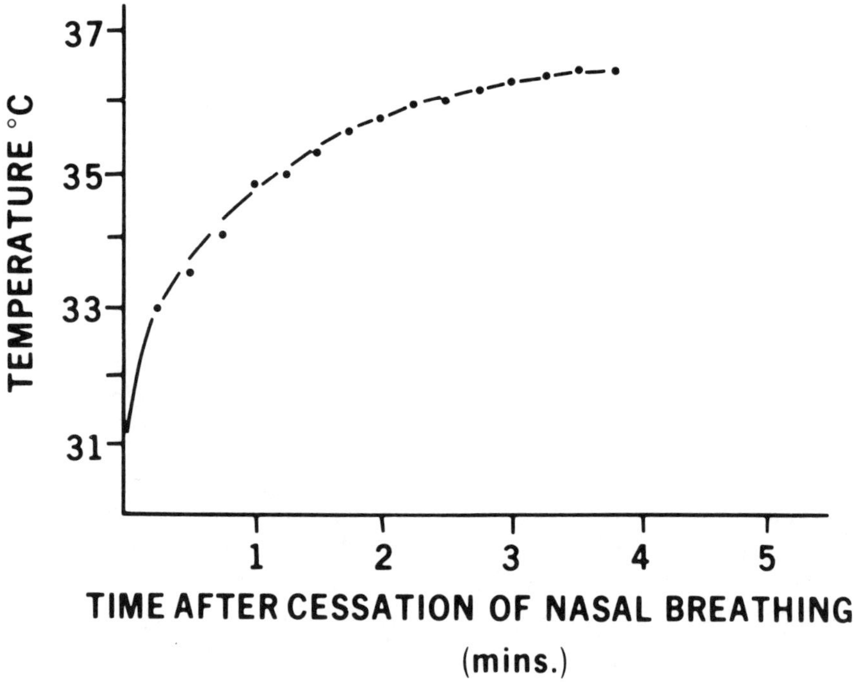

FIG 3–8.
Slow rewarming of turbinate tissues occurs on cessation of nasal breathing. (From Cole P: Respiratory mucosal vascular responses to air conditioning and thermoregulation. *J Laryngol* 1954; 68:613. Used by permission.)

resistance that accompanies breathing cold air (see Chapter 1, "Erectile Mucosa") indicates a response of capacitance vessels; blood content is increased, but measurements have shown that blood flow is reduced, as it is in skin on exposure to cold (Olsson and Bende, personal communication, 1990).[31]

Remote Thermal Stimuli

In addition to the local effect of ambient air on the airway mucosa, warming the skin surface remote from the nose and face increases the temperature of nasal mucosa and of expiratory air, and the converse is found with skin cooling. Furthermore, an increase in whole-body temperature of only 0.5° C in humans results in an increase in nasal expiratory air temperature of 2 to 3° C.[19]

Expiratory air temperatures corresponding with reflex nasal mucosal blood-flow changes in response to skin warming or cooling are paralleled by similar changes in finger temperature and blood flow[19] (Fig 3–9). The extremities of the human body, of which the finger may be regarded as representative, play an important role in heat dissipation and thermoregulation; and, as will be discussed below, it seems that the nasal mucosa behaves in a similar manner.

Moreover, both skin temperature and nasal expiratory air temperature can be changed pharmacologically. Intravenous injection of tolazoline, a peripheral vasodilator, results in an almost immediate increase of several minutes' duration in both skin and nasal expiratory air temperature.[19]

The response to vasoconstrictors and effects on respiratory air temperatures is complicated by the extreme sensitivity of capacitance vessels to α-agonists. In addition to any reduction in blood flow and blood-borne heat,[4] the increase in nasal lumen, resulting from constriction of capacitance vessels, alters the airflow characteristics on which thermal exchanges depend.

Measurements of expiratory air temperature during oral breathing have not shown the responses to thermal stimulation of the skin surface that are manifested during nasal breathing, and generally respiratory

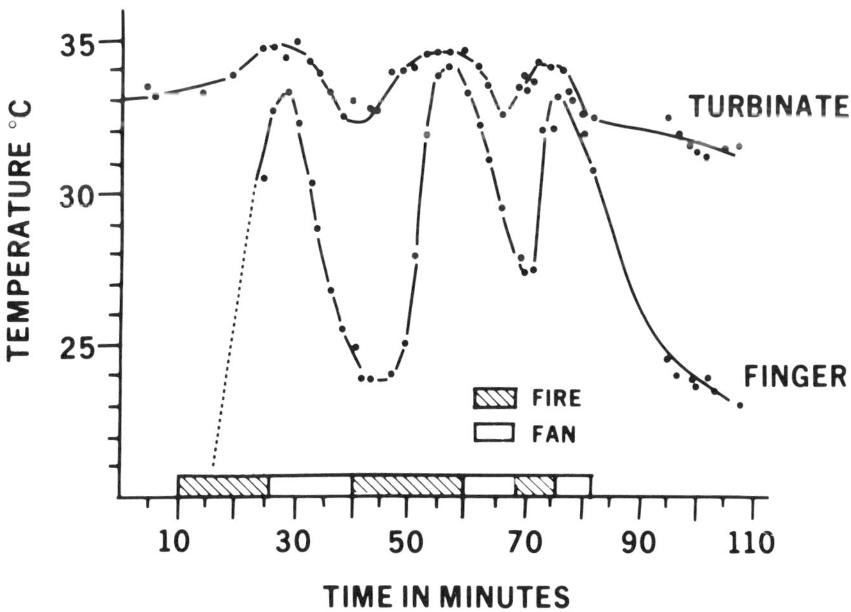

FIG 3–9.

Temperatures reflecting blood flow in finger and nasal mucosa in response to remote thermal stimuli. (From Cole P: Respiratory mucosal vascular responses to air conditioning and thermoregulation. *J Laryngol* 1954; 68:613. Used by permission.)

heat and water losses are greater by the oral route. These human experiments indicate a distinctive function of the nasal mucosa in conditioning expiratory air. It is suggested by the author that this is a vestigial function in man and not usually of great physiologic importance. It is suggested further that this nasal function plays a more crucial role in those animals whose nasal mucosal area is extended in elaborate turbinate structures.

Comparative Animal Studies

Experimental studies with dogs and seals that have extensive turbinates (Fig 3–10; also see Figs 1–1 and 1–2) have shown similar but much more marked changes in nasal expiratory air temperature than humans in response to thermal stimuli to the body surface of comparable intensity. While a moderate skin-chilling stimulus reduces expiratory air temperature of humans from 32° C by 1 to 2° C, a similar stimulus in dogs reduces it several more degrees, from 33° C to as low as 25° C. A warming stimulus has the opposite effect, increasing the expiratory air temperature in humans to 33° C and in dogs to 36° C.

The range of adjustment of nasal expiratory air temperature in response to these thermal stimuli in dogs (11° C) is far greater than in humans (3 to 4° C), and it includes a correspondingly larger adjustment in water content and latent heat of vaporization.[19] It is of interest to note also that the well-insulated, non-sweating dog retains metabolic heat and sustains a raise in body temperature of several degrees with vigorous exercise, then loses much of this heat by panting on recovery from exercise (see also Chapter 2, "Mouth Breathing"). The panting reflex of the dog is very sensitive to thermal stimuli: altering the distance of a moderate heat source (a small electric radiator) from the dog by only a few inches was found to switch the reflex on or off.

There are striking anatomical differences in nasal structures between humans and dogs—indeed, between humans and many animals (see Figs 1–1, 1–2, and 3–10). Non-sweating and well-insulated animals exhibit extensive turbinate structures.[74] Turbinate-surface area of the seal has been calculated to exceed that of its skin, and a sheep's turbinates occupy a nasal volume that exceeds the cerebral capacity of the cranium. Dogs, cats, rabbits, and other furry, non-sweating animals exhibit complex turbinates. Ungulates, which are moderately insulated and can sweat, have turbinates that are intermediate in size and complexity between humans and seals. Humans, who sweat and lack extensive natural insulation, exhibit vestigial turbinate structures.

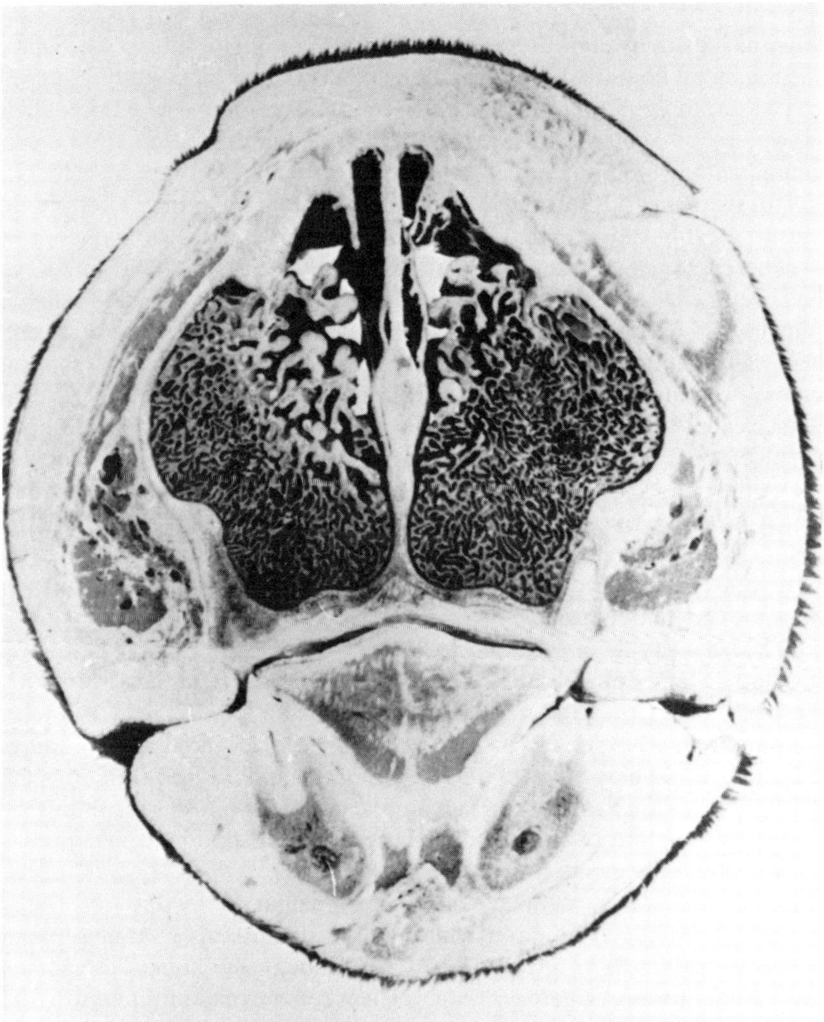

FIG 3–10.
Maxilloturbinate of seal. (From Negus VE: *The Comparative Anatomy and Physiology of the Nose and Paranasal Sinuses.* London, E & S Livingstone, 1958. Used by permission.)

THERMOREGULATION

Turbinate Function

Relationships between the combination of turbinate areas and nasal mucosal blood flow and body insulation and expiratory air condition suggest both a thermoregulatory function and a mechanism for conservation of heat and water.[60, 74] Seals spend several weeks of the mating season ashore, consuming neither food nor drink.[38] It seems reasonable to suppose that complex turbinates and a restricted blood flow through them play a role in the control of expiratory air condition and the conservation of catabolic water.

There are many examples of thermoregulation and heat and water conservation by the air passages that are of significant survival value in animals. The particular importance of these processes to lizards, birds, and small desert animals has been noted.[57] It is reported that desert rats can conserve as much as 90% of the water of expiratory air,[70, 71] and measurements of expiratory air from many other animals have shown effective heat and water recovery. Giraffes recover >60%,[48] seals >70%,[38] and penguins >80%.[58] At a given ambient temperature the reindeer increases its expiratory heat loss very markedly when it has its insulating winter coat.[10] It is suggested that the numerous arteriovenous shunts in the nasal mucosa enable the reindeer to exert a wide range of control of expiratory air temperature.

The recovery figures quoted for these animals would likely be altered substantially and appropriately by extremes of exposure, as has been noted in experiments with humans, dogs, and seals. Their expired heat and water losses would be determined by both local effects of inspired ambient air on temperature and blood flow of the mucosa of the upper respiratory tract and by indirect environmental effects on mucosal vascular reflexes resulting from thermal stimulation of the skin. Together these responses would provide appropriate adjustments of heat and water losses.

Heat and water recovery and thermoregulation by the respiratory passages are relatively unimportant processes for survival of humans in their natural or artificially tropical habitat, but although the human integument is the major thermoregulatory organ, vestiges remain of a turbinate structure and function that is important in many other animals.

SUMMARY

The resistors of the nasal and oral vestibules disrupt the laminar-flow pattern by inducing disturbances in the rapidly moving inspiratory airstream. These disturbances are essential for effective cleansing and conditioning of the air, which takes place by convective transfer and mixing in its brief passage through the large lumen of the upper airways. Increasing thermal demands of ventilation and cold air shift an increasing burden of conditioning to more peripheral airways. The peripheral airways present an enormous mucosal area close to a slowly moving airstream that ensures protection of their terminations from thermal injury, desiccation, and from harmful airborne substances.

Expiratory air returns heat and water to mucosa cooled by inspiration mainly in the nose, where vascular behavior regulates the recovery process appropriately. Regulation of heat and water losses in expiratory air has survival value and is reflected in the elaborate turbinates of many animal species, but both turbinate structure and function are vestigial in humans.

REFERENCES

1. Andersen I, Molhave L: The ambient air, in Proctor DF, Andersen I (eds): *The Nose: Upper Airway Physiology and the Atmospheric Environment.* Amsterdam, Elsevier Biomedical Press, 1982.
2. Andersen I, Lundqvist GR, Jensen PL, et al: Human response to controlled levels of sulfur dioxide. *Arch Environ Health* 1974; 28:31–39.
3. Anderson I, Lundqvist GR, Proctor DF, et al: Human response to controlled levels of inert dust. *Am Rev Respir Dis* 1979; 119:619–627.
4. Andersson K-E, Bende M: Adrenoceptors in the control of human nasal mucosal blood flow. *Ann Otol Rhinol Laryngol* 1984; 3:179–182.
5. Anselmo WT, DeOliveira JAA, Valeri V, et al: Morphology of the human nasal mucosa on the inferior turbinate: A structural model. *Am J Rhinol* 1991; 5(1):11–17.
6. Askenazi J, Silverberg K, Foster R, et al: Effects of breathing apparatus on breathing pattern. *J Appl Physiol* 1980; 48:577–580.
7. Barach AL: Grunting, groaning and pursed-lip breathing. *Bull N Y Acad Med* 1973; 49:666–673.
8. Bartlett D Jr, Remmers JE, Gautier H: Laryngeal regulation of respiratory airflow. *Respir Physiol* 1973; 18:192–204.
9. Beeckmans JM, Shephard RJ: Computer calculation of exercise dead-space. *Respiration* 1971; 28:236–256.
10. Blix AS, Johnsen HK, Mercer JB: On nasal heat exchange and the structural basis for its regulation in reindeer. *Proc Physiol Soc* 1983; (C96):116P.
11. Brain JD: The uptake of inhaled gases by the nose. *Ann Otol Rhinol Laryngol* 1970; 79:529–539.
12. Bruck E: Water in expired air: Physiology and measurement. *J Pediatr* 1962; 60(6):869–881.
13. Cauna N: Blood and nerve supply of the nasal lining, in Proctor DF, Andersen I (eds): *The Nose: Upper Airway Physiology and the Atmospheric Environment.* Amsterdam, Elsevier Biomedical Press, 1982.

14. Clark RE, Orkin LR: Body temperature studies in anesthetized man. *JAMA* 1954; 154(4):311–319.
15. Cockcroft DW: The effect of helium on nasal resistance and nasal flows. *Am Rev Respir Dis* 1979; 120:697–699.
16. Cole P, Forsyth R, Haight JSJ: Respiratory resistance of the oral airway. *Am Rev Respir Dis* 1982; 125:363–365.
17. Cole P: Recordings of respiratory air temperature. *J Laryngol* 1954; 68:295–307.
18. Cole P: Temperature, moisture and heat: Relationships in the upper respiratory tract. *J Laryngol* 1953; 67:449–456.
19. Cole P: Respiratory mucosal vascular responses to air conditioning and thermoregulation. *J Laryngol* 1954; 68:613–622.
20. Cole P: Further observations on conditioning of respiratory air. *J Laryngol* 1953; 67:669–683.
21. Cole P, Forsyth R, Haight JSJ: Respiratory resistance of the oral airway. *Am Rev Respir Dis* 1982; 125:363–365.
22. Cottle MH: Rhino-sphygmo-manometry: An aid in physical diagnosis. *Int Rhinol* 1968; 6:7–26.
23. Dekker E: Transition between laminar and turbulent flow in human trachea. *J Appl Physiol* 1961; 16(6):1060–1064.
24. Dery R, Pelletier J, Jacques A, et al: Humidity in anaesthesiology. *Can Anaesth Soc J* 1967; 14(4):287–297.
25. Ferrus L, Guenard H, Vardon G, et al: Respiratory water loss. *Respir Physiol* 1980; 39:367–381.
26. Forster RE: Diffusion of gases, in *Handbook of Physiology, Section 3, Respiration,* vol 1. Washington, American Physiology Society, 1964.
27. Gautier H, Remmers JE, Bartlett D Jr: Control of duration of expiration. *Respir Physiol* 1973; 18:205–221.
28. Girardin M, Bilgen E, Arbour P: Experimental study of velocity fields in human nasal fossa by laser anemometry. *Ann Otol Rhinol Laryngol* 1983; 92:231–236.
29. Good AL, Sellers AF: Temperature changes in the blood of the pulmonary artery and left atrium of dogs during exposure to extreme cold. *Am J Physiol* 1957; 188:447–450.
30. Gross D, Weiler-Ravell D, Freedman S, et al: Temperature changes within the airways during hyperventilation and exercise. *Chest* 1982; 82:228–232.
31. Hales JRS: Regulation of the cutaneous circulation. *Fed Proc* 1986; 45:2844–2846.
32. Hey EN, Price JF: Nasal conductance and effective airway diameter. *J Physiol* 1982; 330:429–437.
33. Heyden R: Tracheal temperature in laryngectomized patients. *Acta Otolaryngol (Stockh)* 1949; 75:134–137.
34. Heyden R: The respiratory function in laryngectomized patients. *Acta Otolaryngol Suppl (Stockh)* 1950; 85: 1–61.
35. Hinderer KH: Effect of air currents on the naso-pulmonary mucosa. *Rhinology* 1975; 13:1–5.

36. Hirsch JA, Bishop B: Human breathing patterns on mouthpiece or facemask. *J Appl Physiol* 1982; 53(5):1281–1290.
37. Hunt J: *The Conquest of Everest.* New York, EP Dutton, 1954.
38. Huntley AC, Costa DP, Rubin RD: The contribution of nasal countercurrent heat exchange to water balance in the northern elephant seal. *J Exp Biol* 1984; 113:447–454.
39. Hynes B, Silverman F, Cole P, et al: Effects of ozone exposure: A comparison between oral and nasal breathing. *Arch Environ Health* 1988; 43:357–360.
40. Ingelstedt S: Studies on the conditioning of air in the respiratory tract. *Acta Otolaryngol (Stockh)* 1956; 131:1–180.
41. Ingelstedt S: Humidifying capacity of the nose. *Ann Otol Rhinol Laryngol* 1970; 79(3):475–480.
42. Ingelstedt S, Toremalm NG: Airflow patterns and heat transfer within the respiratory tract. *Acta Physiol Scand* 1961; 51:204–217.
43. Ingelstedt S, Toremalm NG: Aerodynamics within the larynx and trachea. *Acta Otolaryngol Suppl (Stockh)* 1960; 158:81–92.
44. Jaeger JJ, Deal EC, Roberts DE Jr, et al: Cold air inhalation and esophageal temperature in exercising humans. *Med Sci Sports Exerc* 1980; 12:365–369.
45. Jaeger MJ, Matthys H: The pattern of flow in the upper human airways. *Respir Physiol* 1969; 6:113–127.
46. Kirkpatrick BM, Sheppard D, Nadel J, et al: Effect of oronasal breathing route on sulfur dioxide-induced bronchoconstriction in exercising asthmatic subjects. *Am Rev Respir Dis* 1982; 124:627–631.
47. Lafortuna CL, Minetti AE, Mognoni P: Inspiratory flow pattern in humans. *J Appl Physiol* 1984; 57(4):1111–1119.
48. Langman VA, Maloiy GMO, Schmidt-Nielsen K, et al: Nasal heat exchange in the giraffe and other large animals. *Respir Physiol* 1979; 37:325–333.
49. Liese W, Joshi R, Cummig G: Humidification of respired gas by nasal mucosa. *Ann Otol Rhinol Laryngol* 1973; 82(3):330–332.
50. Majer EH: Possible vascular regulatory mechanisms in the mucous membrane of the upper respiratory tract. *Acta Otolaryngol (Stockh)* 1968; 65:59–62.
51. Marshall R, Macey DJ: Streamlining of airflow in the upper airways and trachea. *Thorax* 1980; 35:543–545.
52. Mather GW, Nahas GG, Hemingway A: Temperature changes of pulmonary blood during exposure to cold. *Am J Physiol* 1953; 173:390–392.
53. McFadden ER, Pichurko BM, Bowman FH, et al: Thermal mapping of the airways in humans. *J Appl Physiol* 1985; 58(2):564–570.
54. Mead J: Mechanical properties of lungs. *Physiol Rev* 1961; 41:281–330.
55. Melon J, Daele J: La mesure de la permeabilite nasale. *Acta Otolaryngol (Belg)* 1979; 33:643–722.
56. Moritz AR, Weisiger JR: Effects of cold air on air passages and lungs. *Arch Intern Med* 1945; 75:233–240.
57. Murrish DE, Schmidt-Nielsen K: Exhaled air temperature and water conservation in lizards. *Respir Physiol* 1970; 10:151–158.
58. Murrish DE: Respiratory heat and water exchange in penguins. *Respir Physiol* 1973; 19:262–270.

59. Naito K, Cole P, Fraschetti J, et al: Nasal patency: Subjective and objective. *Am J Rhinol* 1989; 3:93–97.
60. Negus VE: *The Comparative Anatomy and Physiology of the Nose and Paranasal Sinuses.* London, Livingstone, 1958.
61. Olson LG, Fouke JM, Hoekje PL, et al: A biomechanical view of upper airway function, in Mathew OP, Sant'Ambrogio G (eds): *Respiratory Function of the Upper Airway.* New York, Marcel Dekker, 1988.
62. O'Neill G, Tolley NS: Theoretical considerations of nasal airflow mechanics and surgical implications. *Clin Otolaryngol* 1988; 13:273–277.
63. Primiano FP Jr, Moranz ME, Montague FW Jr, et al: Conditioning of inspired air by a hygroscopic condenser humidifier. *Crit Care Med* 1984; 8:675–678.
64. Proctor DF: The upper airways: Interface between the lungs and the ambient air, in Settipane GA (ed): *Rhinitis.* Providence, RI, Oceanside Publishing Inc., 1991.
65. Proctor DF, Hardy JB: Studies of respiratory airflow. *Bull Johns Hopkins Hosp* 1949; 85:253–280.
66. Rohrer F: Der Stromungwiderstand in den menschlichen Atemwegen und der Einfluss der unregelmassigen Verzweigung des bronchial Systems auf den Atmungsverlauf in verschiedenen Lungenbezirken. *Arch Ges Physiol* 1915; 162:225–299.
67. Rubenstein E, Pardee RC, Eldridge F: Alveolar-capillary temperature. *J Appl Physiol* 1960; 15(1):10–12.
68. Samzelius-Lejdstrom I: Respiratory movements. *Acta Otolaryngol Suppl (Stockh)* 1939; 35:3–104.
69. Schaefer O, Eaton RDP, Timmermans FJW, et al: Respiratory function impairment and cardiopulmonary consequences in long-time residents of the Canadian Arctic. *Can Med Assoc J* 1980; 123:997–1004.
70. Schmidt-Nielsen K, Hainsworth RF, Murrish DE: Countercurrent heat exchange in the expiratory passages: Effect on water and heat balance. *Respir Physiol* 1970; 9:263–276.
71. Schmidt-Nielsen K: Desert animals, in *Physiological Problems of Heat and Water.* Oxford, Clarendon Press, 1964.
72. Schumacher MJ: Rhinomanometry. *J Allergy Clin Immunol* 1989; 83:711–720.
73. Schumacher MJ, Gaines J, Bescript B: Computer-aided rhinometry: analysis of inspiratory and expiratory nasal pressure-flow curves in subjects with rhinitis. *Comput Biol Med* 1985; 15:187–195.
74. Scott JH: Heat-regulating function of the nasal mucous membrane. *J Laryngol* 1953; 87:461–462.
75. Sedee GA: The relation between the functions of the nose and the lung on the same side of the body. *Int Rhinol* 1969; 7:7–13.
76. Settipane GA: Allergic rhinitis: Update. *Otolaryngol Head Neck Surg* 1986; 94(4):470–475.
77. Silberstein EB, Lewis JT, Quenelle DJ: A study of the physiologic relationship of lower and upper airways with Xenon-133. *Ann Otol Rhinol Laryngol* 1980; 89:62–64.

78. Silverman F: Asthma and respiratory irritants (ozone). *Environ Health Perspect* 1979; 29:131–136.
79. Silverman F, Folinsbee LJ, Barnard J, et al: Pulmonary function changes in ozone: Interaction of concentration and ventilation. *J Appl Physiol* 1976; 41(6):859–864.
80. Swift DL: Physical principles of airflow and transport phenomena influencing air modification, in Proctor DF, Andersen I (eds): *The Nose: Upper Airway Physiology and the Atmospheric Environment.* Amsterdam, Elsevier Biomedical Press, 1982.
81. Swift DL, Proctor DF: Access of air to the respiratory tract, in Brain JD, Proctor DF, Reid LM (eds): *Respiratory Defense Mechanisms.* New York, Marcel Dekker, 1977.
82. Takagi Y, Proctor DF, Salman S, et al: Effects of cold air and carbon dioxide on nasal airflow resistance. *Ann Otolaryngol* 1969; 78:40–48.
83. Thoman RL, Stoker GL, Ross JC: The efficacy of pursed-lips breathing in patients with chronic obstructive pulmonary disease. *Am Rev Respir Dis* 1966; 93(1-3):100–106.
84. Walker JEC, Wells RE, Merrill WE: Heat and water exchange in the respiratory tract. *Am J Med* 1961; 30:259–267.
85. Wit G de: The function of the nose in the aerodynamics of respiration. *Rhinology* 1973; 11:59–67.
86. Woods LDH: The effect of gas physical properties and flow rate on pulmonary ventilation and gas exchange (thesis). Montreal, McGill University, 1974.

SUGGESTED READING

1. Mathew OP, Sant' Ambrogio G (eds): *Respiratory Function of the Upper Airway.* New York, Marcel Dekker, 1988.
2. Proctor DF, Andersen I (eds): *The Nose: Upper Airway Physiology and the Atmospheric Environment.* Amsterdam, Elsevier Biomedical Press, 1982.

CHAPTER 4

Assessment of the Upper Airways

DIAGNOSIS

A Firm Basis for Therapy

Upper-airway diseases causing nasal obstruction and mouth breathing are not of consuming interest to all clinicians; consequently, therapy and follow-up are sometimes halfhearted and results disappointing. Moreover, patients may suffer from a surfeit of therapists. It is not unusual for a child with complaints of a stuffy nose or a chronically open mouth to be under the care of a family practitioner, a pediatrician, an otolaryngologist, an allergist, and an orthodontist, each of whom may harbor the mistaken belief that another practitioner has the tiresome problem in hand. Even with diligent care from all concerned, a successful outcome can be prejudiced by lack of unanimity in diagnosis and in recommendations for management. An adenoidectomy, for example, may seem a matter of greater urgency to an orthodontist than to a pediatrician, and treatment of obstructive adenoid hypertrophy or other airway-obstructive conditions may be postponed by parental indecision. And in many cases, therapeutic decisions are finalized by confused and clinically unqualified parents.

The clinical training and experience of otolaryngologists uniquely equip them to take the bulk of responsibility in the care of patients with diseases of the airways outside the lungs. In addition to the broad range of traditional ENT methods, proficiency in employing recent advances in endoscopy, airflow studies, acoustic reflection, immunology, and imaging extend diagnostic and rational therapeutic possibilities for the otolaryngologist in managing extrapulmonary airway diseases.

SYMPTOMATOLOGY

Nasal Sensation

Sneezing and rhinorrhoea can be assessed from a patient's history or from numbers of sneezes and tissues used as recorded by a patient, but neither the symptom of nasal obstruction nor of the chronically open mouth provides a reliable index of nasal patency or reveals the extent of mouth breathing (see Chapter 2, "Mouth Breathing"). As with other forms of dyspnea, the sensation of impaired nasal breathing depends not only on discrimination of threshold but also on psychologic factors. It has affective and cognitive components.[2] Although some patients may evaluate their nasal patency appropriately, objective measurements compared with an analog symptom scale show that the majority do not.[83] Many identify the side of unilateral obstruction correctly,[51, 52, 79] but it is not unusual to find patients with widely patent nasal airways who complain of nasal stuffiness, even as measurements are being made, and yet others who complain of obstruction of the structurally more patent side.[3] Nor is it unusual for grossly abnormal noses to be found in uncomplaining patients.

Complaints about severity of nasal obstruction show great inter-patient variation and their morphologic basis is not always evident.[20] Objective assessment of nasal patency has shown the inability of healthy subjects to detect marked elevation of nasal resistance induced by aspirin ingestion,[69] and only half those tested were aware of pronounced reduction of nasal resistance resulting from topical application of decongestant (Naito, personal communication, 1991). Indeed, as noted in Chapter 1 under "Nasal Cycle," few healthy subjects are conscious of major physiologic resistance changes that accompany the nasal cycle, recumbent postures, or physical exercise.

Thermal Receptors

The trigeminal nerve supplies sensory branches to the nasal mucosa, but specialized end organs have not been identified (see Chapter 1, "Rhinitis and Turbinate Hypertrophy"). A sensation of chill within the nasal (or oral) cavities is a predominant feature of inspiration; its intensity and penetration increase with airflow velocity, and it is absent in expiration. The sensation is consistent with thermal effects of respiratory airflow. Sensations of both chill and patency are amplified by deep inhalation of ambient air. They are amplified also by inhalation of aromatic substances.[37] Inhalation of the L-menthol isomer vapor and other aromatic substances that contain it are particularly effective in enhancing a sensation of nasal patency, a sensation that is unaccompanied by objective change in airflow resistance. This subjective phenomenon occurred also in half of the subjects who inhaled citronella, an aromatic substance that does not contain menthol.[36] By contrast, passive exposure of healthy subjects to cigarette smoke can give rise to a sensation of nasal stuffiness that is unaccompanied by significant alteration of airflow resistance.[106]

Thermal receptors (or thermoreceptors) are affected by aromatic substances[98] not only in the nasal mucosa but also in skin, as with after-shave preparations. Responses to localized thermal stimuli in humans indicate that receptors abound in the skin of the nasal vestibular region, and nasal sensation suggests they are present also in the caval and nasopharyngeal mucosa,[1, 68] although they have not been identified histologically at any of these sites. Responses indicating the presence of both thermoreceptors and mechanoreceptors in the nasal passages have been demonstrated in the rabbit; the latter receptors adapt rapidly to airflow stimulation.[60] Similar nasal-receptor responses have been reported in the cat.[42] The presence of nasal airflow receptors and of mechanisms remote from the nose that might give rise to sensations of nasal patency or stuffiness have been postulated in humans also. But, apart from auditory perception of nasal or oral airflow, conclusive explanations of the mechanisms of airflow sensation await further elucidation.

In addition to the sensation of nasal airflow, there is evidence to suggest widespread responses to this form of sensory nerve stimulation,[14, 99] which may be of importance to breathing in both awake and sleeping subjects[8, 34, 96, 111] (see Chapter 2, "Breathing in Sleep"). Furthermore, nasal breathing of chilled air reduces the sensation of dyspnea and inhibits respiratory thoracic contraction.[78] These effects are enhanced by increased nasal airflow velocity and diminished by topical anesthesia.[76]

RHINOSCOPY

Subjective Limitations

It has been commented recently by an experienced and respected clinician,[29] with reference to nasal dysfunction, that "few do more than examine the nose in a cursory fashion . . . and there is poor understanding of a group of diseases of which the etiology and therapy are frequently unknown." Nevertheless, diligent rhinoscopy in experienced hands plays an essential and revealing role in ENT examination of patients. However, in many cases, it does not enable the examiner to differentiate with confidence between normal and abnormal, and it has distinct limitations in assessment of nasal patency.[6, 20]

The rigid nasal cavum is unaffected by introduction of a speculum and is capacious by comparison with the valve region. It can accommodate quite prominent swelling, as in response to either topical histamine[47] or simulated septal deviations,[18] and these abnormalities exert relatively little effect on its small airflow resistance (see Figs 1–1 and 1–13 to 1–15). By contrast, the narrow nasal-valve region, which provides the principal resistor of the respiratory tract, is especially vulnerable to obstruction by structural or mucosal abnormality. In the leptorrhine nose, rhinoscopic instrumentation disturbs tissue relationships at this critical site, where simulated swelling of one wall by only a millimeter can produce a major escalation of resistance to respiratory airflow[18, 23, 27] (see Figs 1–13 to 1–15).

Swelling or structural deviation of this degree in the compliant anterior nose cannot be assessed reliably by rhinoscopy but can be readily detected and measured by rhinomanometry.

Discrepancy between results of rhinoscopy and rhinomanometry is an indication for reevaluation. However, it is not uncommon, and statistical analysis has suggested to some observers that the methods might be measuring distinct and independent entities.[51, 70] Furthermore, statistics indicate that, even among experienced clinicians, chance alone could contribute substantially to inter-observer correlations concerning nasal patency.[50]

Anomalous Findings

Anomalous clinical findings from patient history and clinical inspection are frequently encountered by rhinologists. A large proportion of patients complaining of nasal stuffiness are referred to us for objective assessment of nasal patency by practitioners whose clinical examination revealed no evidence of nasal obstruction. In the majority of these cases, despite the patient's prevailing symptoms, rhinomanometry confirms the referring practitioner's findings. Indeed, since symptoms are commonly inconsistent with appearances, criteria required for accurate diagnosis and rational therapy demand critical evaluation and scrupulous judgment.

Since the beginning of this century there have been great advances in rhinologic knowledge, experience, and endoscopic technology; yet, in many cases, rhinoscopic inspection is still as stated in 1914 "incapable of furnishing us with trust-worthy information as to the efficiency of the nasal chambers in performance of their functions . . . statements of patients are still more untrustworthy."[112]

After therapy, too, rhinoscopic and rhinomanometric findings do not always reflect symptomatology.[66, 67] Disappointment, satisfaction, and sometimes surprise may be the result for patients and for clinicians. However, despite their limitations, rhinoscopic assessments of nasal obstruction are more closely correlated with objective measurements of nasal patency than patients' sensations of obstruction.[83]

Clinical comment: The symptom of nasal stuffiness can be misleading to both patient and clinician. Rhinomanometry, which can provide useful support to clinical impressions of patency, can prevent the undertaking of inappropriate therapeutic measures.

OBJECTIVE MEASUREMENT

Rhinomanometry

In view of the subjective nature of a clinician's evaluation and the diagnostic unreliability of symptomatology, it is usually desirable that clinical impressions of nasal patency and of oronasal breathing be supported by objective criteria.[38] Stringent criteria can provide a rational basis for management—and, later, for assessment of therapeutic results.

Transnasal pressure and flow studies, termed *rhinomanometry* by the International Committee on Standardization of Rhinomanometry, provide the most widely used form of objective assessment of nasal patency.[21, 22, 25] These studies have contributed to knowledge of nasal respiratory physiology. They are helpful in appraisal and quality control of therapy, of value in medicolegal documentation, and widely used by allergists in assessing nasal challenges and medications.[80]

Increasingly, an understanding of nasal respiratory pathophysiology enables rhinomanometric techniques to be extended to diagnosis and evaluation of the severity of nasal diseases. Objective airflow findings are dependent on laws of fluid mechanics, a point in favor of their reliability. Certainly methodological errors of rhinomanometry do not exceed in magnitude those of other commonly used laboratory tests.[58] Furthermore, objective methods can reduce the need for large numbers of subjects in clinical trials.[65]

In common with other forms of investigation of dynamic organs, rhinomanometry provides only momentary glimpses of a functional continuum, and results should be appraised with this limitation in mind. The nose is a dynamic organ; spontaneous and induced fluctuations in blood content of erectile tissues are reflected in the constantly changing appearance of the mucosa and in its effects on airflow resistance. It is important to ascertain from patients who complain of nasal obstruction the extent of the sensation as examination and testing are being undertaken—for example, by use of an analog symptom scale—and to enquire about circumstances such as recumbent postures or environmental factors that might initiate or exacerbate a symptom that is absent at the time of examination.

Alternative Objective Methods

Passive rhinomanometry, in which air is drawn or forced through the nose at a controlled rate or pressure, is a practical technique for animal studies. It has been employed also in humans in whom continuous observations can be made and rapid changes in airflow resistance recorded.[104] In a clinical setting, active rhinomanometry is more usual: the patient, seated and at rest, is examined while breathing spontaneously and exclusively through the nose. Many alternative methods are available as well for assessment of nasal patency, several of which are discussed briefly here.[71, 101]

The technique of observing areas of condensation formed by nasal expiration against a *chilled mirror, or other reflecting surface,* has been used in examination of nasal breathing in humans and animals for more than a century.[114] This is a simple method for detecting nasal breathing and demonstrating unilateral obstruction that has also proved useful in following rapid cyclical changes in airflow resistances.[54] Refinements of this method[41] include concentric markings on the condensing surface to aid comparison, and use of a thermographic surface and camera recording.[15]

Peak flowmeters (Wright type) modified for nasal use are employed by several investigators to obtain an index of nasal patency. The instruments are simple in construction, inexpensive, and readily portable.[105] They are particularly convenient for unaided patient use and for frequently repeated measurements. Disadvantages include effort dependence and variability of results,[59] but further development of sniff testing by this method has promise of improved precision.[92]

Strip chart recording of transnasal pressure and/or flow along a time axis as a means of assessing nasal patency has a lengthy and respected history, but it is less used today than formerly.[32] By means of this method, the tracings or measurements of inspiratory and expiratory amplitude and duration are inspected to detect nasal abnormality and to monitor therapy. The technique has been superseded in most centers by pressure and flow recordings, but the time scale of the earlier method provides additional information. Obstructive nasal-airway abnormalities are detected by time-scale recordings, and the possible relationship between waveform and nasal sensation can be examined (Chapter 2, "Mouth Breathing"). Transnasal pressure-time and flow-time recordings have complex origins and reflect functions and dysfunctions remote from the nose; in fact, effects of cardiac abnormalities have even been ascribed to characteristics of the tracings.[33, 81]

Oscillometry has been used sporadically to determine nasal resistance. A loudspeaker provides sinusoidal sound-wave oscillations, which are superimposed on the breathing cycle. Impedance of the respiratory airways is measured from pressure and flow signals as the oscillator is applied to nose and mouth, and nasal resistance is calculated from the difference. Digital signal processing might enable this technique to be more widely exploited.[72]

Recent developments in rhinometry include extension of *acoustic-reflection* techniques to the nasal airways (Fig 4–1; see also Fig 1–5). These methods, which have been used for several years in investigation of the

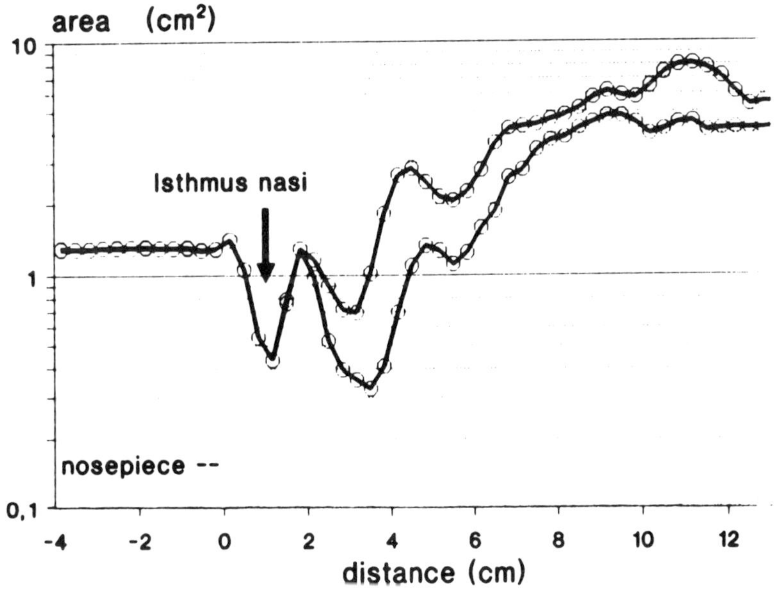

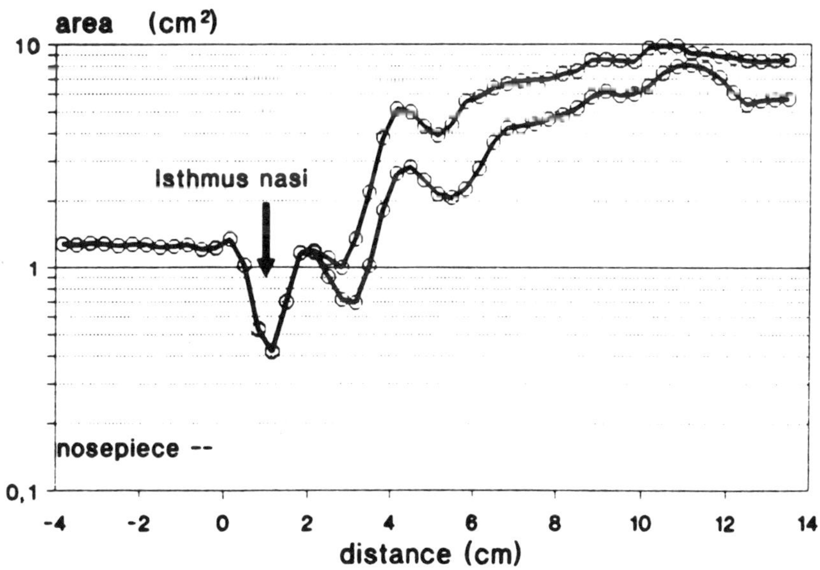

FIG 4–1.

Acoustic-reflection studies before and after inferior turbinate reduction. (From Lenders H, Persig W: Diagnostic value of acoustic rhinometry: Patients with allergic and vasomotor rhinitis compared. *Rhinology* 1990; 28:5. Used by permission.)

geometry of the tracheal, laryngeal, and pharyngeal airways,[57] have clearly displayed airway narrowing of the nasal valve and changes in size of the inferior turbinates in response to topical applications and to surgical reductions.[55, 75]

Results of acoustic rhinometry are reproducible and consistent with tomographic imaging, with measurements by water-volume displacement, and with rhinomanometry. Septal deviations and intranasal tumors have been demonstrated, and assessments of adenoid volume have shown close agreement with the volume of tissues removed by adenoidectomy. A distinct advantage of acoustic rhinometry over imaging studies and rhinoscopy is its ability to measure dimensions of an orifice independently from its obliquity since it is in the sound path of the acoustic signal.[46] This may account for the relatively high values of valve cross section that have been obtained by this method compared with other measurements.[7, 94] Furthermore, measurements by acoustic reflection entail minimal disturbance of the patient. A single snapshot of nasal geometry can be obtained in an instant or the airway can be observed continuously. In addition to its undoubted experimental usefulness, this promising technique may well find an important place in the clinician's armamentarium.

INDICES OF NASAL PATENCY

Values Derived From Pressure and Flow

There are many alternative indices of nasal patency. Of the several parameters that can be derived from transnasal pressure and flow studies, resistance to respiratory airflow is among the most widely accepted (Table 4–1). The International Committee on Standardization of Rhinomanometry (ICSR)[19] recommends the determination of resistance from concomitant measurements of transnasal pressure and flow of respiratory air. These measurements are obtained during exclusive and spontaneous nasal breathing in subjects at rest and are expressed as a ratio ($Rn = \mathrm{K}\, P/\dot{V}$) in Pa/cm^3/sec (cms H_2O/L/sec $\times$ 1/10). The ratios can be obtained from rectangular or polar coordinates of a predetermined point or points on the transnasal pressure-flow curve (see following discussion).

Alternatives to resistance as a measure of patency have their advocates, most with convincing reasons and, in some cases, for specialized investigations. Of the patency values derived from transnasal pressure and flow (see Tables 4–1 and 4–2), a hydrokinetic equation and resulting hydraulic cross-sectional area is reported to be less pressure- or flow-dependent than

TABLE 4–1.
Alternative Determinants of Nasal Patency*†

Areas of condensation
Anemometry:
Hot-wire
Thermocouple
Thermistor
Acoustic
Nasopharyngeal pressure
Maximum inspiratory or expiratory $\dot{V}$
Pressure and flow derivatives:
ΔP at fixed $\dot{V}$
$\dot{V}$ at fixed ΔP
Work $\Delta P \times V$
Power $\Delta P \times \dot{V}$
Resistance $\Delta P/\dot{V}$
Conductance $\dot{V}/\Delta P$
Cross-sectional area
Log transforms

*$\dot{V}$ = Flow; V = volume; ΔP = differential pressure.
†Resistance and conductance can be measured at *i* = designated point in the $\Delta P/\dot{V}$ curve; *ii* = peak values; *iii* = computer averaged; *iv* = different exponents of $\dot{V}$ between 1 and 2.

TABLE 4–2.
Computed Respiratory Parameters*†

Minute volume	
Frequency	
Tidal volume	
Duration	Measured in inspiration, expiration, and complete breaths (applies to Duration through R_n computer-averaged)
Average $\dot{V}$	
Peak $\dot{V}$	
Average ΔP	
Peak ΔP	
Work	
Power	
Hydraulic cross-section	
R_n at 100 Pa	
R_n at 150 Pa	
R_n computer-averaged	

*Inspiratory, expiratory, and total
†$\dot{V}$ = Flow; ΔP = differential pressure; R_n = nasal resistance; Pa = pascals.

resistance.[30, 95, 107] In order to simplify comparison of results from different investigators, it is desirable that, where possible, alternative preferences of individual investigators be accompanied by patency values expressed in accordance with ICSR recommendations.

x-y Recordings

Nowadays, in most rhinological centers, x-y recordings are used to assess nasal patency (see Fig 3–3). Customarily the recordings are obtained electronically from pressure transducers and flow-measuring devices of appropriate sensitivity and frequency response. Computerized plots of transnasal pressure against flow are displayed on-line by means of a monitor or an oscilloscope, and as a further convenience, digitization of the signals can enable computerized processing of pressure and flow data to compute several nasal and other respiratory variables, like those shown in Table 4–2, for display, storage, or hard copy. Different indices of patency can be obtained simultaneously by this technique, and stored data may be retrieved for further processing and statistical analysis at the convenience of the investigator.

The transnasal pressure-flow curve (see Fig 3–3 and accompanying discussion in Chapter 3) is typically sigmoid in shape and, although its amplitude may vary, its course remains remarkably consistent over a lengthy series of breaths in an individual subject. The differing curves obtained from a large number of subjects cross only at the origin and can be arranged in radial order,[10, 11] each curve representing a different resistance to nasal respiratory airflow as obtained at the time of testing. Since an individual subject's pressure-flow curve is rotated toward the pressure axis by nasal obstruction and toward the flow axis by an increase in patency, the ratio of coordinates of a predetermined point or points on the curves of different subjects can be used to express their individual indices of patency.[10, 11]

Artifacts

Not all investigators who use coordinate methods choose the same predetermined point of pressure or flow, but with computer assistance, different indices can be obtained simultaneously.[103] In Scandinavia, polar coordinates and predetermined radii are used. The 100 Pa point is a common compromise, widely accepted as a standard in Japan. However, many patients at rest (both Asian and white) do not achieve as high a transnasal pressure as 100 Pa during spontaneous nasal breathing through combined nasal cavities.[87] In such cases slight hyperventilation may achieve the designated differential pressure—but hyperventilation is not entirely without risk, since it can alter the pressure-flow curve.

Hyperventilation extends the extremities of the curve notably in the expiratory phase, which is sometimes attenuated in subjects breathing spontaneously at rest (see Chapter 3, "Flow Characteristics"). The main course of the curve usually remains unchanged, but in some cases the whole curve is rotated toward the pressure axis by marked increases in ventilation (Auger et al., unpublished, 1990; see Fig 3–4). In these cases, since inspiratory and expiratory limbs of the curve are affected, whole-curve rotation occurs independently from transmural pressure effects on alar positioning. In addition to whole-curve rotation, transmural pressures that increase with ventilation could affect cross-sectional dimensions and resistances of the compliant valve region and introduce asymmetry between limbs of the curve. Furthermore, hyperventilation of only a few breaths increases nasal airflow resistance by promoting congestion of erectile tissue (see Chapter 1, "Erectile Mucosa").

Application of respiratory equipment to a subject's airway alters the pattern of breathing and increases ventilation,[4, 56] and it is probable that, in many cases, it is this response to a face mask or nasal nozzle that augments tidal flow sufficiently to generate transnasal pressures in excess of 100 Pa and promote symmetry of the pressure-flow tracings. Ventilation artifacts are less likely to result from the relatively noninvasive plethysmographic methods. Seventy-five Pa (or "radius 1" in the Scandinavian Brom's method) is probably a more practical transnasal pressure point for measurement of flow and calculation of resistance than the higher values that are commonly employed.

Increased ventilation can elevate resistances calculated at a predetermined point, at peak points, and by averaging. However, standardization of breathing, which has been suggested as a strategy for overcoming dependence of patency values on breathing pattern, is not easy to attain, and the need to establish appropriate parameters for age and size complicate this approach further.

Despite the artifacts (see also "Objective Assessment of Pharyngeal Airway" later in this chapter) and sources of disagreement that have been discussed, peak pressure and flow points that are used by some observers to calculate resistance[79] produce results that do not differ greatly from 100 Pa values. Also, resistance of the whole pressure-flow curve can be averaged by digital sampling at 50 Hz or faster throughout one or several breathing cycles.[22] In subjects breathing spontaneously at rest, similar values are obtained by all three methods over a range of resistances that extend to 0.4 Pa/cm^3/sec, a value that is well beyond that found in the combined cavities of healthy adult noses.[82] The latter two methods offer an additional advantage in not requiring a designated pressure or flow point for calculation of resistances. For clinical assessments in our own laboratories, we measure averaged resistance by 50-Hz sampling during spontaneous breathing in resting subjects and record also resistances at 100 Pa and 150 Pa, if these levels are achieved, and also at peak levels. The computer program includes the option to display and print both graphics and the text parameters shown in Table 4–2, together with coefficients of variation. It also allows manipulations of stored raw digital data.

In addition to differences in breathing pattern and in methods of calculation, differences in measuring techniques can affect transnasal pressure and flow and derived values. Techniques most commonly used are discussed here for readers who may be interested in such technical details.

Transnasal Pressure Measurement

Transnasal pressures (Fig 4–2) are measured by the following three methods:

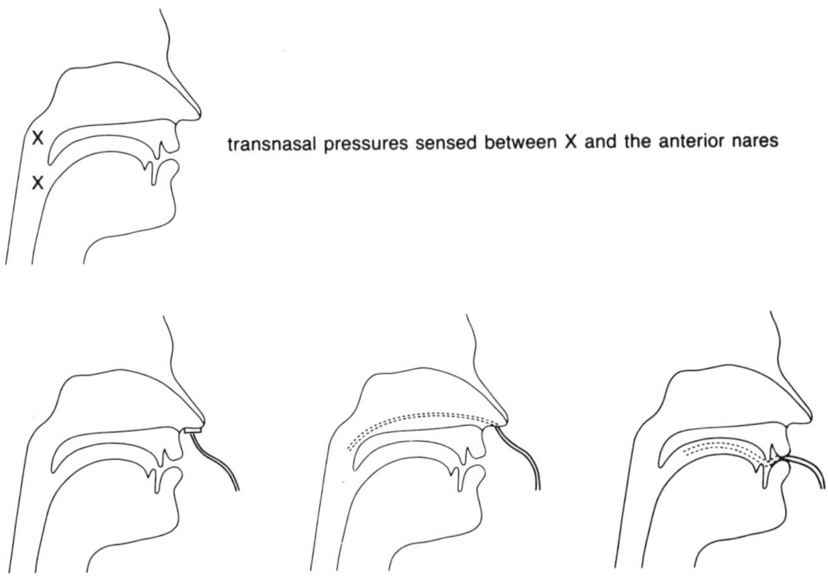

anterior nasal catheter (corresponding naris sealed opposite side patent)

per nasal catheter to nasopharynx

per oral catheter to oropharynx

FIG 4–2.

Transnasal pressure determination.

1. A peroral tube passed between closed lips toward the oropharynx
2. A fine pernasal tube passed along the floor of the nose to the nasopharynx
3. A fine tube sealed in a nasal vestibule as the opposite nasal cavity remains patent.

Method 1: Posterior Rhinomanometry

In the method of posterior rhinomanometry, both palatoglossal and palatopharyngeal airways must remain patent while pharyngeal pressures are measured through the peroral tube, and respiratory air flows exclusively through nose and pharynx. The majority of subjects perform this maneuver spontaneously. Assistance can be obtained by feedback from observation of a monitor screen. Few fail if persistance, patience, and persuasion are exercised by subject and examiner. Indeed, acceptable results have been obtained from children as young as 3½ years, and the success rate of a skilled technician exceeds by far the 50% to 70% frequently quoted in the literature.[91] This method is of particular value in children, since it includes the nasopharyngeal airway and can detect obstruction by lymphoid tissues in this region.

Method 2: Pernasal Technique

The pernasal technique requires an 8F-gauge infant feeding tube (or similar tube). It is lubricated with lidocaine gel and passed 8 cm along the floor of a nasal cavity to the nasopharynx. Any slight discomfort ceases as soon as the tube is immobilized and secured to the upper lip with adhesive tape. The lateral opening at the tip of the tube must remain directed vertically to avoid occlusion by mucosa. Many subjects have tolerated the tube in situ for several hours (e.g., during sleep studies) without irritation, but an occasional patient responds to insertion with increased airflow resistance and mucus secretion in the intubated nasal cavity. This is uncommon, and the risk of it occurring is minimized by promptness in insertion and fixation of the tube as well as in taking measurements. The pernasal technique has fewer demands on cooperation by the patient than posterior rhinomanometry and is less time-consuming. It is used mainly in adults since measurements do not include the nasopharyngeal airway that may be of particular interest in pediatric patients.

Method 3: Anterior Rhinomanometry

Anterior rhinomanometry, like the pernasal technique, also requires minimal patient cooperation but suffers the disadvantage of excluding the nasopharyngeal airway. Measurements from the two nasal cavities are separated by the time interval between removal and replacement of the pressure-detecting tube and face mask. Reliability of calculations of combined resistance by application of Ohm's Law for parallel resistors is vulnerable to vascular fluctuations of the nasal mucosa with consequent resistance fluctuations during this interval[23, 35] (Fig 4–3). Furthermore, redisplacement of facial tissues by replacement of the mask risks resistive consequences.

Substantial unilateral vascular fluctuations in resistance can take place in only a few moments[53] (see Figs 1–26 and 1–27), but they are abolished by application of a topical decongestant that enables matching results to be obtained by anterior and posterior rhinomanometry[23, 24] (see Fig 4–3 again). Additional disadvantages of the anterior method include the unnatural mode and increased airflow velocity of unilateral breathing, differences in

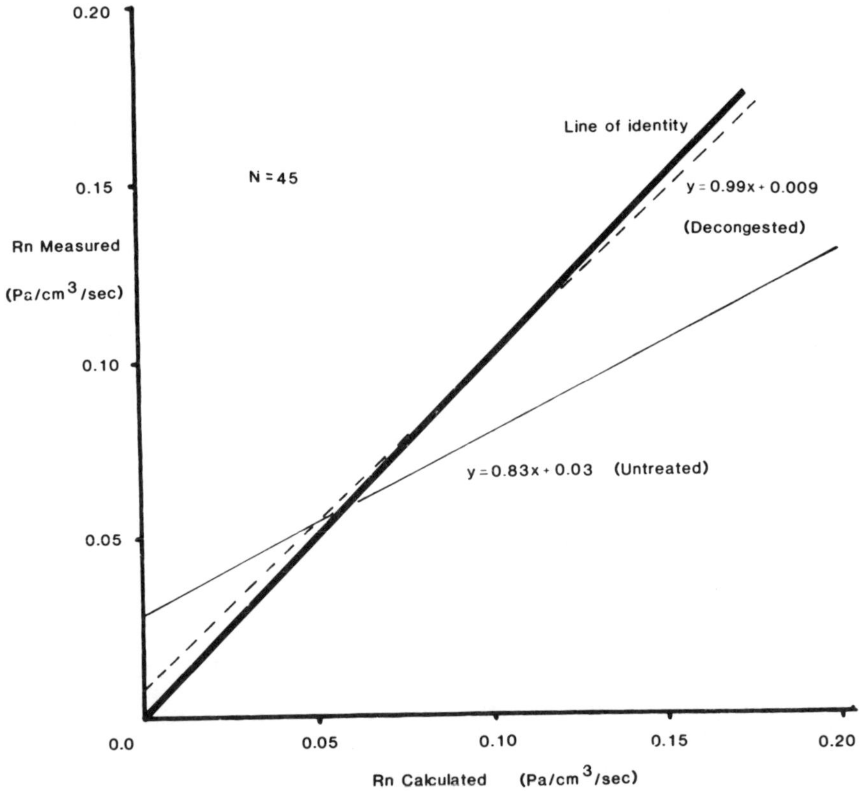

FIG 4–3.

Anterior and posterior rhinomanometry in untreated and decongested noses compared. Decongested measurements lie on line of identity. (From Cole P, Ayiomamitis A, Ohki M: Anterior and posterior rhinomanometry. *Rhinology* 1989; 27:257. Used by permission.)

breaths between the two sides, and the risk of alar compliance with transmural respiratory pressures. The latter risks are possibly increased by inhibition of alar dilator muscle activity in response to contralateral vestibular occlusion. Most artifacts tend to increase resistance values.

Anterior rhinomanometry is widely accepted as adequate for clinical purposes and is probably the most commonly used method. Errors are minimized when the labile vascular mucosa is stabilized by decongestant (see Figure 4–3) and a well-chosen mask is applied with care. It should be stressed in the instruction of technicians that whatever method is employed, every precaution must be taken in the use of all measuring devices to avoid distortion of compliant tissues about the anterior nose, the primary resistive site of the respiratory airways.

Transnasal Airflow Measurement

As with transnasal pressure measurement, several different methods are employed for measuring transnasal airflow. The equipment usually includes a laminar-flow element or other flow-measuring device incorporated with one of the following:

1. A nozzle inserted in a nasal vestibule
2. A face mask that incudes the nose
3. A head-out displacement-type of body plethysmograph that measures whole-body respiratory volume change
4. An inductive plethysmograph that measures respiratory body-volume change electronically without a laminar-flow element

Method 1: Insertion of a Nozzle

Inserting a nozzle is a convenient method, but airflow resistance of the nozzle must be minimized, and there is a high risk that the process of securing an air-seal between nozzle and nostril can cause dilation or distortion of the compliant nasal valve, resulting in major resistive consequences at this most resistive segment of the respiratory airways. Reliable measurements can be obtained only by exercise of extreme care in choice and application of the nozzle.

Method 2: Face Masking

Face masking is the most common method. Choice of mask is important in order to achieve an air-seal between mask and face with minimal discomfort and minimal distortion of facial tissues. Displacement of mobile facial tissues as far from the nostrils as the zygomatic region can affect nasal airflow resistance substantially.[23] Leaks between face and mask increase pressure-flow (resistance) values but, despite careful application, forceful pressure of the mask against the face to ensure an air-seal increases the risk of nasal vestibular distortion and resistive consequences. In our experience, full face masks (firefighter type) and modified CPAP nasal masks have proved the most reliable. SCUBA and anesthetic masks have been found to increase both magnitude and variability of nasal resistances significantly as compared with a head-out body plethysmograph that leaves the face and nostrils entirely free from interference.

Method 3: Displacement Plethysmograph

The head-out displacement-type of body plethysmograph with a low-resistance laminar-flow element (150 cm^2 400 mesh nylon laboratory filter) incorporated in its side wall is an excellent method. It may appear cumbersome and rather formidable by comparison with a mask or a nozzle, but it is a rugged, reliable, and stable apparatus. The pressure-flow ratio is linear across the flow element with this method, and the frequency response is adequate for respiratory maneuvers.[45] Moreover, calibration is simple and infrequently required.[84] We check the complete system weekly with a piston pump and resistor that mimic nasal breathing, and recalibrate for clinical assessments if variation from previous measurements is $>5\%$.

The plethysmograph box can be constructed inexpensively from ¾-inch laminated particle board, and specifications are not very demanding. The method enables the face and the nasal and oral orifices of the subject to remain entirely free from interference and available for observation, video studies, electromyograms, alar retraction, nose/mouth breathing, and so on, while measurements of spontaneous or other forms of breathing at rest or with exercise are conducted.[85, 86] By contrast with a face mask, the plethysmograph easily accommodates subjects of all shapes and sizes in comfort, leaks are not a problem, and children are entertained rather than intimidated by it.

Method 4: Inductive Plethysmography

Inductive plethysmography is an attractively noninvasive method. The author's experience with this form of measurement is limited to its use as an indicator of thoracic and abdominal respiratory volume change in sleeping subjects. Inductive vests, which quantitatively assess volume change of a cylinder from alterations in its circumference,[110] have been used successfully by other investigators[109] to determine thoracic and abdominal volume change and thus to determine respiratory airflow.

CLINICAL RHINOMANOMETRY

The Toronto Experience

Practical diagnostic rhinomanometric sequences of resistance measurements shown in Table 4–3 reflect our Toronto experience with more than 15,000 subjects. Examples of normal and pathologic adult values are tabulated.[22]

In the Toronto upper-airway investigation laboratories, where the nasal airways of more than 2,000 patients are investigated annually, nasal resistances are determined from airflow measurements obtained by means of a head-out body plethysmograph, and transnasal pressures are measured via a pernasal (adults) or peroral (children) tube. In field work we use a face mask for airflow measurement in place of the more cumbersome plethysmograph and a peroral tube for pressures. In both situations digitized pressure and flow signals are processed by computer.

Establishment of the upper limits of resistance values presented in Table 4–3 results more from a combination of experience and intuition than from statistical treatment of data. Lower limits are less definitive, but if they are one half or less of the quoted upper limits, they arouse suspicion of abnormality.

In addition to the many factors that influence pressure and flow indices of patency, population studies show that results of resistance measurements are skewed toward higher values, and parametric statistics are unsuitable for

TABLE 4–3.
Clinical Examples of Rhinomanometric Results: Nasal Airflow Resistances (Pa/cm³/sec)

	Diagnosis*			
	A*	B*	C*	Guidelines*
Untreated				
Both sides	0.210	0.365	0.247	<0.25
Left	0.398	1.690	0.438	Varies with cycle
Right	0.499	0.496	0.996	Varies with cycle
Decongested				
Both sides	0.135	0.097	0.243	<0.10
Left	0.255	0.308	0.350	<0.4
Right	0.349	0.222	0.956	<0.4
Retracted				
Left	0.117	0.140	0.147	<0.2
Right	0.183	0.068	0.171	<0.2

*A = unremarkable findings; B = mucovascular disease; C = right anterior fixed obstruction; Guidelines = Indicate approximate adult upper limits.

comparisons of raw data. Logarithmic transforms normalize resistance values and, unlike customary resistance measurements, conductance (the reciprocal of resistance) does not extend toward infinity as obstruction increases, and it also provides a more normalized distribution of data.[44, 49, 90] Conductance is an example of a useful alternative index of patency.

Other Centers

Our results are in general agreement with published figures from other centers, but minor dissimilarities exist among centers. Several investigators report obtaining resistance values at a transnasal reference pressure of 150 Pa, and they are 25% to 30% greater than values obtained at 100 Pa. As a further example, the convenient and widely employed alternative method of anterior rhinomanometry produces results that frequently differ from those obtained by direct posterior rhinomanometry. Application of Ohm's Law for parallel resistors to unilateral resistance values only approximates the combined resistance of both nasal cavities measured simultaneously.[35] Factors that contribute to the discrepancy have been discussed previously in this chapter.

Diagnostic Decongestant

Several observers have noted that although the increased nasal patency that follows application of a topical decongestant demonstrates a mucovascular component of airflow resistance (see Table 4–3), it does not exclude the presence of a structural contribution to obstruction. Considerable relief of obstruction from either mucosal or structural causes can be obtained by decongestant in many cases. The head-out plethysmograph is convenient for measurements from separate decongested nasal cavities with and without alar retraction for determination of the magnitude and location of structural obstruction as demonstrated in Table 4–3.

Other Problems With Rhinomanometry

In addition to problems of differences in technique and in indices of patency that have been discussed above, there are other problems with rhinomanometry. For example, do measurements obtained from subjects breathing spontaneously at rest best represent obstructive pathology and symptomatology, or would they be better taken during a specified pattern or patterns of breathing frequency and tidal flow? Another question is whether nasal respiratory maneuvers can be developed to detect and quantitate alar dysfunction?[31] Furthermore, is there an index of nasal patency or other type of measurement better correlated with symptomatology than resistance? These problems have yet to be resolved.

OBJECTIVE ASSESSMENT OF ORONASAL BREATHING

An Adjunct to Rhinomanometry

In addition to the importance of quantitative evaluation of nasal-airway patency in diagnosis and management of upper-airway obstructive diseases, quantitative assessment of oronasal distribution of respiratory airflow is a desirable objective. As discussed in Chapter 2 under "Mouth Breathing," neither the extent of lip separation nor the degree of nasal patency indicate to the examining clinician the proportion of respiratory airflow that passes through a patient's mouth.[74] Objective methods are required to quantitate the abnormality and the results of therapy. It has been shown by these methods that a decrease in the oral fraction of respiratory air of a "mouth breather"[73] accompanies increased nasal patency resulting from application of a topical decongestant. These results demonstrate a measurable therapeutic benefit of improved nasal patency. Certainly, critical assessment of other therapeutic results would be strengthened by greater use of objective tests.

Invasive techniques of measurement can disturb the labile balance and behavioral overlay that determine spontaneous distribution of respiratory airflow between oral and nasal airways.[43] In an attempt to minimize this artifact, minimally invasive equipment consisting of a head-out body plethysmograph and a comfortable, modified CPAP nasal mask have been employed.[73, 74] Digitized flow signals from mask and plethysmograph with the use of a computer enable the breathing pattern to be displayed and its stability monitored. When stability is established, a data-acquisition computer program is activated and computed data are displayed and stored. Hard copy of nasal and oral airflow values during inspiration and expiration over a series of consecutive breaths can be produced.

Reassurance of the patient by a friendly and informal atmosphere, distraction of attention from the measuring devices by an entertaining video, and provision of comfortable equipment contribute toward minimizing physiologic and psychologic disturbances. Consistency and reproducibility of results suggests that these measures are effective. Other investigators have taken advantage of the noninvasive inductive plethysmographic method[109] for this type of objective assessment of oronasal breathing, and both lines of investigation are adding information that contributes to our understanding of oronasal breathing and its associated abnormalities.

OBJECTIVE ASSESSMENT OF THE PHARYNGEAL AIRWAY

In Wakefulness and Sleep

Lateral X-ray and cephalometry are employed to assess the dimensions of the soft tissues of the tongue and palate and the pharyngeal airspace and to determine relationships between bony points of the skull base, face, mandible, and hyoid. In some centers this information is regarded as being of cardinal diagnostic importance, but one must remember that these are two-dimensional studies of a three-dimensional situation. Influences of posture, breathing, and swallowing on mobility and positioning of the soft tissues must also be considered.[40]

Fluoroscopy and computed tomography have also been employed in awake and sleeping patients but are not in general use. Acoustic reflection is used mainly in a research setting.[39] An acoustic signal is generated and projected into the airways via the mouth. Intensities and timing of the reflected signal enable a computerized display of a plot of cross-sectional dimensions of the airway at different sites.[57] Pharyngeal airspace and compliance have been evaluated by acoustic reflection as diagnostic measures in apneic patients[9, 12, 13] and in the assessment of UPPP results.[113]

Respiratory airflow pressures have been measured at different sites in the pharynx by means of open catheters, balloon catheters, and transducer-tipped catheters (Millar type) inserted pernasally in awake and sleeping subjects,[17, 62, 63] and these results are discussed in Chapter 2 under "Breathing in Sleep" and "Snoring."

Airflow resistances can be obtained by adding a flow-measuring device to the pressure-detecting system to enable signal and data processing to be performed electronically as described in rhinomanometry. Indeed, pressure and flow studies similar to those described for investigation of respiratory function of the nose and mouth are currently employed in awake and sleeping subjects to explore these same parameters in the pharynx and its subdivisions, and also in the laryngeal and tracheobronchial airways.[28a]

NASAL AIRWAY STABILITY

Variation Over Time

Changes in physiologic and pathologic mucosal status are reflected in nasal airflow–resistance changes that are amplified in structurally narrowed airway segments. Nevertheless, over time, resistances and work of nasal breathing[21, 24, 25, 28] of combined healthy nasal cavities of individual subjects at rest remain remarkably stable in the absence of strong disturbing stimuli (Fig 4–4). A sensation of nasal stuffiness (see above) may result from exposures to moderate degrees of mechanical irritation, nose blowing, ambient temperature or humidity, and concentrations of ozone, sulfur dioxide, and cigarette smoke[106] that are commonly encountered. But these exposures exert surprisingly little effect[28] on baseline nasal resistances as determined by objective measurement (see "Symptomatology" earlier in this chapter). Indeed, repeated rhinomanometric assessments demonstrate that coefficients of intra-subject variation in resistance of the combined nasal cavities of healthy individuals approximate only 10%/hour, 12%/day and

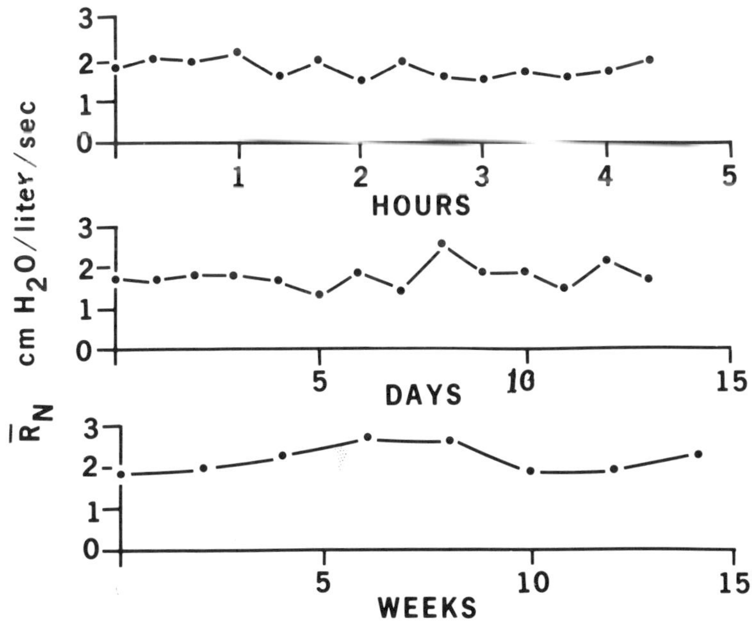

FIG 4–4.

Stability of resistance over time of the combined nasal cavities. (From Cole P, Fastag O, Forsyth R: Variability in nasal resistance measurements. *J Otolaryngol* 1980; 9:309. Used by permission.)

< 20% over a period of months. These measurements were made in young adults breathing spontaneously, at rest, in a comfortable environment; and variability was decreased further when noses were decongested.[24, 25, 28, 104]

Variation With Age

Healthy children show greater inter-subject variation than adults. Also, nasal resistances of many young children fall within the adult range, although mean and median resistances of large groups are negatively correlated with age[61, 91, 93, 97, 108] (Figs 4–5 and 4–6). Transnasal respiratory differential pressures in neonates are not very different from those in adults, but calculation of resistances from their small tidal flows results in values that exceed those of adults by a factor approaching 10.[102] Adult values are

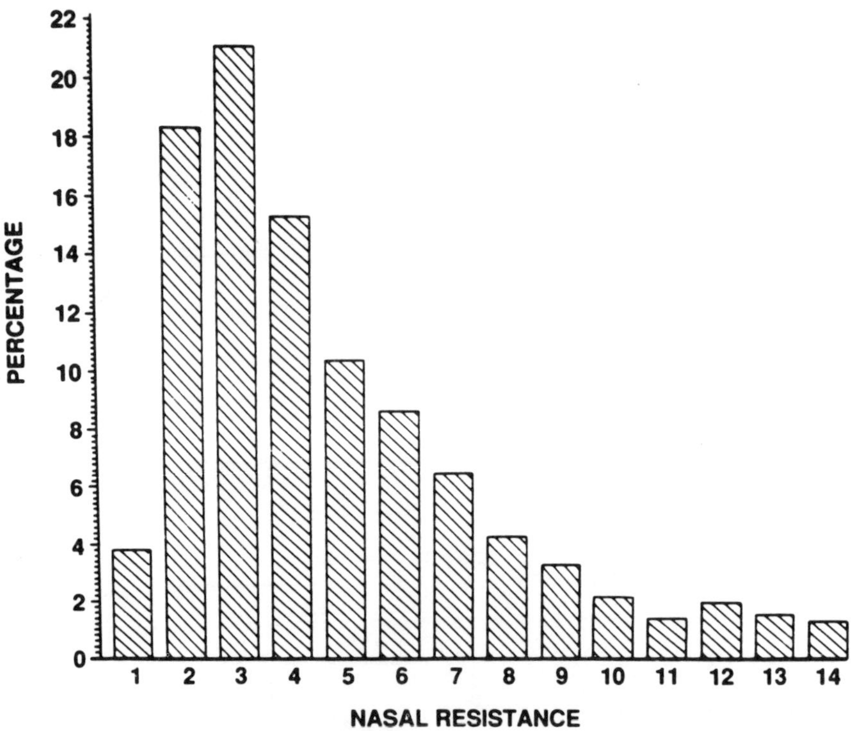

FIG 4–5.

Nasal resistances of 1,000 subjects aged 4 to 18 years. (From Parker LP, Crysdale WS, Cole P, et al: Rhinomanometry in children. *Int J Pediatr Otorhinolaryngol* 1989; 17:127. Used by permission.)

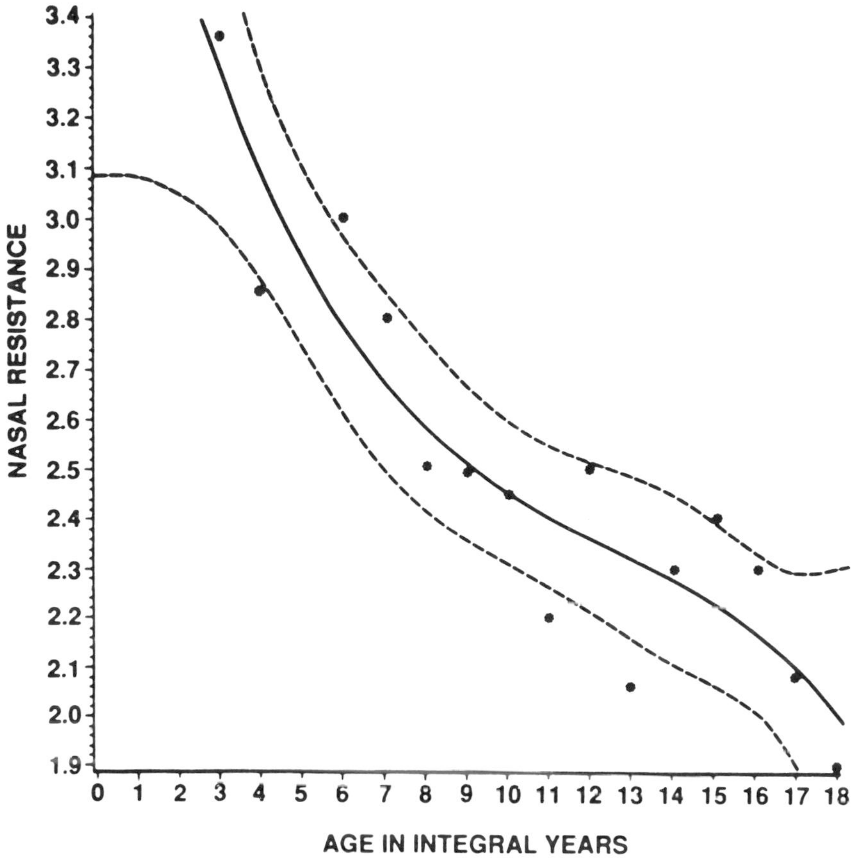

FIG 4–6.

Correlation of nasal resistance with age (95% confidence limits). (From Parker LP, Crysdale WS, Cole P, et al: Rhinomanometry in children. *Int J Pediatr Otorhinolaryngol* 1989; 17:127. Used by permission.)

attained in the mid-teens. In one study, 20 octagenarians averaged a nasal resistance at the lower end of the normal range shown in Table 4–3 (Cole and Haight, unpublished, 1985).

Variation With Race

Several investigators have noted marked racial differences in nasal dimensions, and corresponding airflow resistances have been obtained by posterior rhinomanometry in Canadian residents of different races.[89]

TABLE 4–4.
Measurements of Nostril Dimensions (mm)*

	White (N = 24)	Asian (N = 20)	Black (N = 17)	Statistics
Width of nose	34.0 ± 2.6	38.7 ± 1.9	42.5 ± 3.8	$P<.05$
Dorsal-Ventral (A)	14.8 ± 1.9	10.4 ± 1.5	10.8 ± 1.7	NS
Transverse (B)	9.8 ± 1.7	10.6 ± 2.0	12.6 ± 4.2	NS
A-B	5.0 ± 2.4	−0.2 ± 1.6	−3.3 ± 2.8	$P<.05$

*From Ohki M, Naito K, Cole P: Dimensions and resistance of the human nose: Racial differences. *Laryngoscope* 1991; 101(3):276. Used by permission.

TABLE 4–5.
Measurement of Nasal Resistance (Pa/cm³/sec)*

	White (N = 24)	Asian (N = 20)	Black (N = 17)	Statistics
Untreated both NR	0.184 ± 0.052	0.146 ± 0.046	0.129 ± 0.054	$P<.05$
Untreated unilateral NR	0.485 ± 0.223	0.406 ± 0.171	0.338 ± 0.189	$P<.05$
Decongested both NR	0.127 ± 0.034	0.109 ± 0.030	0.077 ± 0.020	$P<.05$
Decongested unilateral NR	0.298 ± 0.104	0.254 ± 0.093	0.194 ± 0.071	$P<.05$

NR = Nasal resistance.

*From Ohki M, Naito K, Cole P: Dimensions and resistances of the human nose: Racial differences. *Laryngoscope* 1991; 101(3):276. Used by permission.

Leptorrhine noses (mostly found in the white race) were found to be most resistive, Asian less so, and platyrrhine black noses the least (Tables 4–4 and 4–5; also see Fig 1–9). Greater platyrrhine nasal resistances are reported from measurements obtained by anterior rhinomanometry in Nigeria,[5] but a comparison of resistances between white, black, and Hispanic noses in Texas showed insignificant interracial differences.[16]

Consequences of Erectile Tissue Changes

Resistive consequences of spontaneous (e.g., cyclical) and induced (e.g., by posture or body-surface pressures) changes in nasal erectile tissues are not all trivial; moreover, they can be quite rapid and are often reciprocal[48, 64] (see Figs 1–26 and 1–27). Unilateral measurements show frequent and apparently spontaneous resistance changes in healthy noses, and it appears that there are resistive fluctuations of short duration superimposed on the more sluggish course of the nasal cycle. They are most marked in the more congested side of the nose, where the resistive effects of slight changes in mucosal dimensions are amplified by small dimensions of the residual airway; but these fluctuations exert only a small effect on total nasal resistance. Although frequency of the nasal cycle is measured in hours, the switch between phases is often rapid—it can occupy minutes only—and, as discussed above, any of these rapid changes can upset the Ohm's Law calculations that are used in anterior rhinomanometric assessments of total nasal resistance (see Fig 4–3).

Also, as already mentioned (Chapter 1, "Erectile Mucosa"), decongestion by exercise can be even more rapid than by topical decongestant and equally intense. Hyperventilation, cold inspiratory air, and irritants produce the opposite effect. But, with the exception of some cases of nasal allergy where post-exercise rebound congestion occurs,[88] nasal vascular responses are usually short-lived on cessation of the stimulus, and resistances return to pre-stimulus level within minutes (see Fig 1–19). Nevertheless, it is prudent to precede diagnostic rhinomanometry by a 30-minute period during which the patient is seated comfortably at rest in an innocuous environment, a period that can be usefully occupied with documentation, history taking, and clinical examination.

In addition to the physiologic and pathologic responses already described, there are many systemic diseases[100] and medications[77] that exert vasoactive effects on nasal capacitance vessels and therefore must be considered by the clinician in assessing nasal-airway patency.

> **Clinical comment:** Respiratory airflow resistance of the combined nasal cavities of the healthy nose remains stable unless disturbed by strong local or remote stimuli, by vasoactive medications, or by local—or, in some cases, systemic—diseases. Unilateral resistances are more labile.

SUMMARY

The well-trained and experienced otolaryngologist should take the leading role in management of upper-airway diseases. It is imperative to keep in mind the limitations of subjective assessments of nasal patency and oronasal breathing by patient and clinician. Objective methods provide additional information that can be clinically useful, but these results, too, must be evaluated with discernment. Despite their limitations, compliance with recommendations of the International Committee on Standardization of Rhinomanometry is recommended in order to facilitate comparison among results obtained by different investigators. Post-therapeutic results deserve at least as much critical assessment as that devoted to diagnosis.

Resistances of healthy adult noses remain stable over time despite exposure to common ambient irritants. Resistances of childrens' noses vary more widely, are greater on average, and approach adult values in the mid-teens. Objective airflow studies in awake and sleeping patients are of great clinical and pathophysiologic importance to the advancement of knowledge and thus to diagnosis, treatment, and follow-up of nasal, oral, and pharyngeal disorders of respiratory function.

REFERENCES

1. Aldren C, Tolley NS: Further studies on nasal sensation of airflow. *Rhinology* 1991; 29(1):49–55.
2. Altose M, Cherniak N: Respiratory sensations and dyspnea. *J Appl Physiol* 1985; 58(4):1051–1054.
3. Arbour P, Kern EB: Paradoxical nasal obstruction. *Can J Otolaryngol* 1975; 4:333–338.
4. Askenazi J, Silverberg P, Foster R, et al: Effects of breathing apparatus on breathing pattern. *J Appl Physiol* 1980; 48:577–580.
5. Babatola FDO: Nasal resistance values in the adult negroid Nigerian. *Rhinology* 1990; 28:269–273.
6. Bachmann W, Nieder TH: Der kliniche Wert der Rhinomanometrie. *Laryngol Rhinol* 1978; 57:379–383.
7. Bachmann W, Legler U: Studies on the structure and function of the anterior section of the nose by means of luminal impressions. *Acta Otolaryng (Stockh)* 1972; 73:433–442.
8. Basner RC, Ringler J, Berkowitz S, et al: Effect of inspired air temperature on genioglossus activity during nose breathing in awake humans. *J Appl Physiol* 1990; 69(3):1098–1103.
9. Bradley TD, Brown IG, Grossman RF: Pharyngeal size in snorers, non-snorers and patients with obstructive sleep apnea. *N Engl J Med* 1986; 315:1327–1331.
10. Broms P: Rhinomanometry (thesis), 1980; University of Lund, Sweden.
11. Broms P, Jonson B, Lamm CJ: Rhinomanometry II. A system for numerical description of nasal airway resistance. *Acta Otolaryngol (Stockh)* 1982; 94:157–168.
12. Brown IG, Bradley TD, Phillipson EA, et al: Pharyngeal compliance in snoring subjects with and without obstructive sleep apnea. *Am Rev Respir Dis* 1985; 132:211–215.
13. Brown IG, McClean PA, Boucher R, et al: Changes in pharyngeal cross-sectional area with posture and application of continuous positive pressure in patients with obstructive sleep apnea. *Am Rev Respir Dis* 1987; 136:628–633.

14. But VI, Klimova-Cherkasova VI: Afferent fibers from the upper respiratory tract in branches of the trigeminal nerve. *Byulleten Eksperimental noi Biologii i Meditsini* 1967; 64(12):13–16.
15. Canter RJ: A non-invasive method of demonstrating the nasal cycle using flexible liquid crystal thermography. *Clin Otolaryngology* 1986; 11(5):329–336.
16. Calhoun KH, House W, Hokanson JA, et al: Normal nasal airway resistance in noses of different sizes and shapes. *Otolaryngol Head Neck Surg* 1990; 103(4):605–609.
17. Chaban R, Cole P, Hoffstein V: Site of upper airway obstruction in patients with idiopathic obstructive sleep apnea. *Laryngoscope* 1988; 98:641–648.
18. Chaban R, Cole P, Naito K: Simulated septal deviations (2). *Arch Otolaryngol Head Neck Surg* 1988; 114:413–415.
19. Clement PAR: Committee report on standardization of rhinomanometry. *Rhinology* 1984; 22:151–155.
20. Clement PAR, Hirsch C: Rhinomanometry: A review. *ORL J Otorhinolaryngol Relat Spec* 1984; 46:173–191.
21. Cole P: Rhinomanometry 1988: Practice and trends. *Laryngoscope* 1989; 99(3):311–315.
22. Cole P: Toronto rhinomanometry: Laboratory, field and clinical studies. *J Otolaryngol* 1988; 17;331–335.
23. Cole P, Naito K, Chaban R, et al: Unilateral and bilateral nasal resistance. *Rhinology* 1988; 26:209–216.
24. Cole P, Ayiomamitis A, Ohki M: Anterior and posterior rhinomanometry. *Rhinology* 1989; 27:257–262.
25. Cole P: Stability of nasal airflow resistance. *Clin Otolaryngol Allied Sciences* 1989; 14:177–182.
26. Cole P: Nasal patency and its assessment. *Am J Rhinology* 1987; 1:135–139.
27. Cole P, Chaban R, Naito K, et al: The obstructive nasal septum: effect of simulated deviated deviations on nasal airflow resistance. *Arch Otolaryngol Head Neck Surg* 1988; 114:410–412.
28. Cole P, Fastag O, Forsyth R: Variability in nasal resistance measurements. *J Otolaryngol* 1980; 9(4):309–315.
28a. Cole P, Savand P, Miljeteig H, et al: Resistances in respiratory airflow of the extrapulmonary airways. *Laryngoscope* 1992 (in press).
29. Connell JT: Objective measurements of nasal airflow and other diagnostic nasal tests. *Clin Rev Allergy* 1984; 2:213–223.
30. Connell JT: An instrument for measuring effective cross-section of the nasal airway. *J Allergy* 1966; 37(3):127–134.
31. Corvera G, Corvera J, Ayora MF: Rhinometria computarizada. *Arch Invest Med (Mex)* 1985; 16:275–281.
32. Cottle MH: Rhino-sphygmo-manometry: An aid in physical diagnosis. *Int Rhinol* 1968; 6:7–26.
33. Cottle MH: Nasal breathing pressures and cardio-pulmonary illness. *Eye Ear Nose Throat Mon* 1972; 51:331–340.
34. Douglas NJ, White DP, Weil JV, et al: Effect of breathing route on ventilation and ventilatory drive. *Respir Physiol* 1983; 51:209–218.

35. Dvoracek JE, Hillis A, Rossing RG: Comparison of sequential anterior and posterior rhinomanometry. *J Allergy Clin Immunol* 1985; 76:577–582.
36. Eccles R: Effects of menthol on nasal sensation of airflow, in Green BG, Mason JR, Kare MR (eds): *Irritation. Chemical senses,* vol 2. New York, Marcel Dekker, 1990.
37. Eccles R, Lancashire B, Tolley NS: Experimental studies on nasal sensation of airflow. *Acta Otolaryngol (Stockh)* 1987; 103:303–306.
38. Eiser N: The hitch-hikers guide to nasal airway patency. *Repir Med* 1990; 84:179–183.
39. Fredberg JJ, Wohl MV, Glass GM, Dorkin HI: Airway area by acoustic reflections measured at the mouth. *J Appl Physiol* 1980; 48:749–758.
40. Fujita S: Surgical treatment of obstructive sleep apnea, in Guilleminault C, Partinen M (eds): *Obstructive Sleep Apnea Syndrome: Clinical Research and Treatment.* New York, Raven Press, 1990.
41. Gertner R, Podoshin L, Fradis M: A simple method for measuring the nasal airway in clinical work. *J Laryngol Otol* 1984; 98:351–355.
42. Glebovsky VD, Bayev AV: Stimulation of nasal cavity mucous trigeminal receptors with respiratory airflows. *Sechenov Physiol J USSR* 1984; LLX:1534–1541.
43. Gleeson K, Zwillich CW, Braier K, et al: Breathing route during sleep. *Am Rev Respir Dis* 1986; 134:115–120.
44. Gordon ASD, McCaffrey TV, Kern EB, et al: Rhinomanometry for preoperative and postoperative assessment of nasal obstruction. *Otolaryngol Head Neck Surg* 1989; 101:20–26.
45. Griffin PM, Zamel N: Volume-displacement body plethysmograph using a large flowmeter without pressure compensation. *J Appl Physiol* 1979; 47:1127–1130.
46. Grymer LF, Hilberg O, Pedersen O, et al: Acoustic rhinometry: Values from adults with subjective normal nasal patency. *Rhinology* 1991; 29(1):35–47.
47. Haight JSJ, Cole P: The site and function of the nasal valve. *Laryngoscope* 1983; 93(1):49–55.
48. Haight JSJ, Cole P: Is the nasal cycle an artifact? The role of asymmetrical postures. *Laryngoscope* 1989; 99(5):538–541.
49. Hamilton LH: Effect of xylometazoline nasal spray on nasal conductance in subjects with coryza. *J Otolaryngol* 1981; 10(2):109–116.
50. Hardcastle PF, Haake von N, Murray JAM: Observer variation in clinical examination of the nasal airway. *Clin Otolaryngol* 1985; 10:3–7.
51. Hardcastle PF, White A, Prescott RJ: Clinical and rhinometric assessment of the nasal airway—do they measure the same entity? *Clin Otolaryngol* 1988; 13:185–191.
52. Hardcastle PF, White A, Prescott RJ: Clinical or rhinometric assessment of the nasal airway—Which is better? *Clin Otolaryngol* 1988; 13:381–385.
53. Hasegawa M, Kern EB, O'Brien PC: Dynamic changes of nasal resistance. *Ann Otol Rhinol Laryngol* 1979; 88:66–71.

54. Havas TE, Cole P, Gullane PJ, et al: The nasal cycle after laryngectomy. *Acta Otolaryngol (Stockh)* 1987; 103:111–116.
55. Hilberg AC, Swift DL, Pedersen OF: Acoustic rhinometry: Evaluation of nasal cavity geometry by acoustic reflection. *J Appl Physiol* 1989; 66(1):295–303.
56. Hirsch JA, Bishop B: Human breathing patterns on mouthpiece or facemask. *J Appl Physiol* 1982; 53(5):1281–1290.
57. Hoffstein V, Fredberg JJ: The acoustic reflection technique for non-invasive assessment of upper airway area. *Eur Respir J* 1991 (in press).
58. Holmstrom M, Kumlien J: A clinical follow-up of septal surgery. *Clin Otolaryngol* 1988; 13:115–120.
59. Holmstrom M, Scadding GK, Lund VJ, et al: Assessment of nasal obstruction. A comparison between rhinomanometry and nasal inspiratory peak flow. *Rhinology* 1990; 28(3):191–196.
60. Hoshino T: In vitro electrophysiologic studies on nasal airway receptors of the rabbit. *Ann Otol Rhinol Laryngol* 1988; 97:294–297.
61. Hoshino T, Togawa K, Nishihira S: Statistical analysis of changes of pediatric nasal patency with growth. *Laryngoscope* 1988; 98:219–225.
62. Hudgel DW: Variable site of narrowing among obstructive sleep apnea patients. *J Appl Physiol* 1986; 61(4):1403–1409.
63. Hudgel DW, Hendricks C: Palate and hypopharynx: Sites of inspiratory narrowing of the upper airway during sleep. *Am Rev Respir Dis* 1988; 138:1542–1547.
64. Hudgel DW, Robertson DW: Nasal resistance during wakefulness and sleep in normal man. *Acta Otolaryngol (Stockh)* 1984; 98:130–135.
65. Hynes B, Cole P, Forte V, et al: The evaluation of intranasal topical beclomethasonespray in the treatment of children with non-purulent rhinitis using rhinometric, cytologic and symptomatologic assessment. *J Otolaryngol* 1989; 18(4):151–154.
66. Jessen M, Ivarsson A, Malm M: Nasal airway resistance and symptoms after functional septoplasty: Comparison of findings at 9 months and 9 years. *Clin Otolaryngol* 1989; 14:231–234.
67. Jessen M: Nasal obstruction: An epidemiologic and rhinomanometric evaluation (thesis), 1989; University of Lund, Malm, Sweden.
68. Jones AS, Wight RG, Durham LH: The distribution of thermoreceptors within the nasal cavity. *Clin Otolaryngol* 1989; 14:235–239.
69. Jones AS, Lancer JM, Shone GR, et al: The effect of aspirin on nasal resistance to airflow. *BMJ* 1985; 290:1171–1173.
70. Jones AS, Willat DJ, Durham LM: Nasal airflow resistance and sensation. *J Laryngol Otol Rhinol* 1989; 103:909–911.
71. Jones AS, Viani L, Phillips D, et al: Objective assessment of nasal patency. *Clin Otolaryngol* 1991; 16:206–211.
72. Landser FJ, Nagels J, van der Woestijne KP: Implementation by means of a microprocessor technique for the measurement of total respiratory impedance during spontaneous breathing. *Prog Respir Res* 1979; 11:135–143.

73. Leiberman A, Ohki M, Cole P: The open mouth and oro-nasal breathing. *Am J Rhinol* 1991; 5(1):1–5.
74. Leiberman A, Ohki M, Forte V, et al: Nose/mouth distribution of respiratory airflow in "mouth breathing" children. *Acta Otolaryngol (Stockh)* 1990; 109:454–460.
75. Lenders H, Persig W: Diagnostic value of acoustic rhinometry: Patients with allergic and vasomotor rhinitis compared. *Rhinology* 1990; 28(1):5–16.
76. Liss HP, Grant BJB: The effect of nasal flow on breathlessness in patients with chronic obstructive pulmonary disease. *Am Rev Respir Dis* 1988; 137:1285–1288.
77. Mabry RL: Nasal stuffiness due to systemic medications. *Otolaryngol Head Neck Surg* 1983; 91(1):93–94.
78. McBride B, Whitelaw WA: A physiological stimulus to upper airway receptors in humans. *J Appl Physiol* 1981; 51(5):1189–1197.
79. McCaffrey TV, Kern EB: Clinical evaluation of nasal obstruction: A study of 1000 patients. *Arch Otolaryngol* 1979; 105:542–545.
80. McLean JA: Rhinomanometry and experimental nasal challenge, in Settipane GA (ed): *Rhinitis.* Providence, RI, OceanSide Publishing Inc., 1991.
81. Montserrat-Viladieu JM: Rhinometry in cardiac infarction. *Rhinology* 1977; 15:25–31.
82. Naito K, Cole P, Chaban R, et al: Computer averaged nasal resistance. Rhinology 1989; 27:45–52.
83. Naito K, Cole P, Chaban R, et al: Nasal resistance, sensation of obstruction and rhinoscopic findings compared. *Am J Rhinol* 1988; 2(2):65–69.
84. Niinimaa V, Cole P, Mintz S, et al: A head-out body plethysmograph. *J Appl Physiol* 1979; 47:1336–1339.
85. Niinimaa V, Cole P, Mintz S, et al: Oronasal distribution of respiratory airflow. *Respir Physiol* 1981; 43:69–75.
86. Niinimaa V, Cole P, Mintz S, et al: The switching point from nasal to oronasal breathing. *Respir Physiol* 1980; 42:61–71.
87. Ohki M, Hasegawa M: Studies of transnasal pressure and airflow values in a Japanese population. *Rhinology* 1986; 24:277–282.
88. Ohki M, Hasegawa M, Sakuma A: Exercise-induced nasal obstruction in patients with allergic rhinitis. *Am J Rhinol* 1989; 3(1):1–4.
89. Ohki M, Naito K, Cole P: Dimensions and resistances of the human nose: Racial differences. *Laryngoscope* 1991; 101(3):276–278.
90. Pallanch JF, McCaffrey TV, Kern EB: Normal nasal resistance. *Otolaryngol Head Neck Surg* 1985; 93:778–785.
91. Parker LP, Crysdale WS, Cole P, et al: Rhinomanometry in children. *Int J Pediatr Otorhinolaryngol* 1989; 17:127–137.
92. Pertuze J, Watson A, Pride NB: Maximum airflow through the nose in humans. *J Appl Physiol* 1991; 70(3):1369–1376.
93. Principato JJ, Wolf P: Pediatric nasal resistance. *Laryngoscope* 1985; 95:1067–1069.

94. Proctor DF: The upper airway, in Proctor DF, Andersen I (eds): *The Nose: Upper Airway Physiology and the Atmospheric Environment.* Amsterdam, Elsevier Biomedical Press, 1982.
95. Riveron RP: Cross-sectional area as a measure of nasal resistance. *Rhinology* 1990; 28:257–264.
96. Rubin AH, Phillipson EA, Lavie P: The effect of airway anesthesia on breathing in sleep. *Chest* 1983; 84(3):337.
97. Saito A, Nishihata S: Nasal airway resistance in children. *Rhinology* 1981; 19:149–154.
98. Schafer K, Braun HA, Isenberg C: Effect of menthol on cold receptor activity. Analysis of receptor activity. *J Gen Physiol* 1986; 88:757–776.
99. Servit Z, Kristof M, Strejckova A: Activating effect of nasal and oral hyperventilation on epileptic electrographic phenomena: Reflex mechanisms of nasal origin. *Epilepsia* 1981; 22:321–329.
100. Settipane GA: Nasal manifestations of systemic diseases, in Settipane GA (ed): *Rhinitis.* Providence, RI, OceanSide Publishing Inc., 1991.
101. Shelton DM, Pertuze J, Gleeson MJ, et al: Comparison of oscillation with three other methods of measuring nasal airways resistance. *Respir Med* 1990; 84:100–106.
102. Solow B, Pietersen B: Nasal airway resistance in the newborn. *Rhinology* 1991; 29(1):27–33.
103. Sulsenti G, Palma P: Sviluppi in rinomanometria. Rinomanometro computerizzato con maschera elettronica integrata. *Il Valsalva* 1989; 65(2):92–103.
104. Syabbalo NC, Bundgaard A, Entholm P, et al: Measurement and regulation of nasal airflow resistance in man. *Rhinology* 1986; 24:87–101.
105. Taylor G, MacNeil AR, Freed DLJ: Assessing the degree of nasal patency by measuring peak expiratory flow rate through the nose. *J Allergy Clin Immunol* 1973; 52:193–198.
106. Urch RB, Silverman F, Corey P, et al: Does suggestibility modify acute reactions to passive cigarette smoke exposure? *Environ Res* 1988; 47:34–47.
107. Warren DW, Hairfield WM, Seaton DL, et al: The relationship between nasal airway cross-sectional area and nasal resistance. *Am J Orthod Dentofacial Orthop* 1987; 92:390–395.
108. Warren DW, Hairfield WM, Dalston ET: Effect of age on nasal cross-sectional area and respiratory mode in children. *Laryngoscope* 1990; 100:89–93.
109. Warren DW, Hinton VA, Hairfield WM: Measurement of nasal and oral respiration using inductive plethysmography. *Am J Orthod* 1986; 89:480–484.
110. Watson H: The technology of inductive respiratory plethysmography. Presented at the 3rd International Symposium of Ambulatory Monitoring 1979; Clinical Research Centre, Harrow, London, England.
111. White DP, Cadieux RJ, Lombard RM, et al: The effects of nasal anesthesia on breathing during sleep. *Am Rev Respir Dis* 1985; 132:972–975.

112. Wright J, Smith H: *A Textbook of the Diseases of the Nose and Throat.* Philadelphia, Lea & Febiger, 1914.
113. Wright S, Haight JSJ, Zamel N, et al: Changes in pharyngeal properties after uveopalatopharyngoplasty 1989; 99:62–65.
114. Zwaardemaker H: Ademmaanslag al diagnosticum der nasal stenose. *Ned Tijdschr Geneeskd* 1889; 25:297–300.

Index